Bone-Building/ Body-Shaping Workout

Strength, Health, Beauty

in Just 16 Minutes a Day!

Joyce L. Vedral, Ph.D.

A FIRESIDE BOOK
Published by Simon & Schuster

Fireside
Rockefeller Center
1230 Avenue of the Americas
New York, NY 10020

FIRESIDE and colophon are registered trademarks
of Simon & Schuster Inc.

Book design by Richard Oriolo
Bodywear provided by Dance France
Photography by Don Banks
Hair and makeup by Pam Arnone
Gym Shoes by Reebok International

Manufactured in the United States of America

10 9 8 7 6 5 4

Library of Congress Cataloging-in-Publication Data
Vedral, Joyce L.
    Bone-building/body-shaping workout : strength, health, beauty in
just 16 minutes a day! / Joyce L. Vedral.
      p.   cm.
    "A Fireside book."
    Includes bibliographical references and index.
    1. Exercise for women.   2. Physical fitness for women.   3. Beauty,
Personal.   I. Title.
RA778.V426   1998
613.7'045—dc21   98-14428
                                                            CIP

ISBN 0-684-84731-0

To all the women of the future who realize that
working out with light weights the right
way is truly the fountain of youth!

Acknowledgments

To Roz Siegel, my talented editor, for your enthusiasm and belief in this project and your continual willingness to go the extra mile.

To Mel Berger of William Morris Agency for being ever present and for your willing input.

To Cherylynne Li for your fresh ideas regarding the cover of this book and for your calm, pleasant, intelligent demeanor.

To Don Banks of Don Banks Photography, New York, for your cheerful, creative photography—both for the cover and the inside photographs.

To Pam Arnone for doing a wonderful job on the hair and makeup, both for the cover and inside photographs.

To Dance France for providing all the workout clothing—cover and interior.

To Ken's Fitness Center in Farmingdale, Long Island, for providing a wonderful place to work out—baby-sitting services included—for those women who wish to use a fitness center.

To 24-Hour Fitness Centers in Las Vegas, Nevada, and all over the United States for providing a wonderful workout environment (baby-sitting included) and to manager Becky Most for your kind and sensitive willingness to help people.

To Kathy Harris and Michelle Simms, my fit friends who are true "amigos." I love you both.

To Joe and Betty Weider who started it all!

To the women who have requested this book. This one's for you.

Contents

Foreword

As a board-certified family care practitioner with a focus on female health, especially osteoporosis, it gives me great pleasure to see the *Bone-Building/Body-Shaping Workout* come into existence because in it women of every age will find a realistic, time-efficient way to not only prevent loss of bone density and muscle strength but also *increase* both!

I am delighted to see Joyce Vedral emphasizing that women in their twenties and thirties should begin resistance training to solidify their "bone base" and that she also offers a realistic, simple, easy-to-do-at-home workout which can be done by women, whether they have exercised before or not, in their forties, fifties, sixties, and older.

What I like most about this book is its emphasis on the most vulnerable fracture points—with exercises specifically targeted to build bone-supporting muscle and bone in those areas. Merely working out with weights is not enough: One must systematically challenge each body part in isolation. This workout does exactly that.

In addition to the above, this clearly illustrated system will result, in many ways, in a reversal of the aging process: better posture, more energy, improved balance and strength (so important for various sports), toned, defined muscles, and an in-built method of keeping weight down as a woman ages.

Bone-Building/Body-Shaping Workout provides an excellent way for beginners to start—with a time investment of only eight to sixteen minutes a day—and allow a gradual buildup to thirty-two-minute workouts. Vedral wisely advises that women check with their doctors before starting this or any workout! With that in mind, I say go to it! This one is for all of us.

Alesia J. Wagner, D.O.
Medical Director
Total Family Care
N. Las Vegas, Nevada

Bone-Building/ Body-Shaping Workout

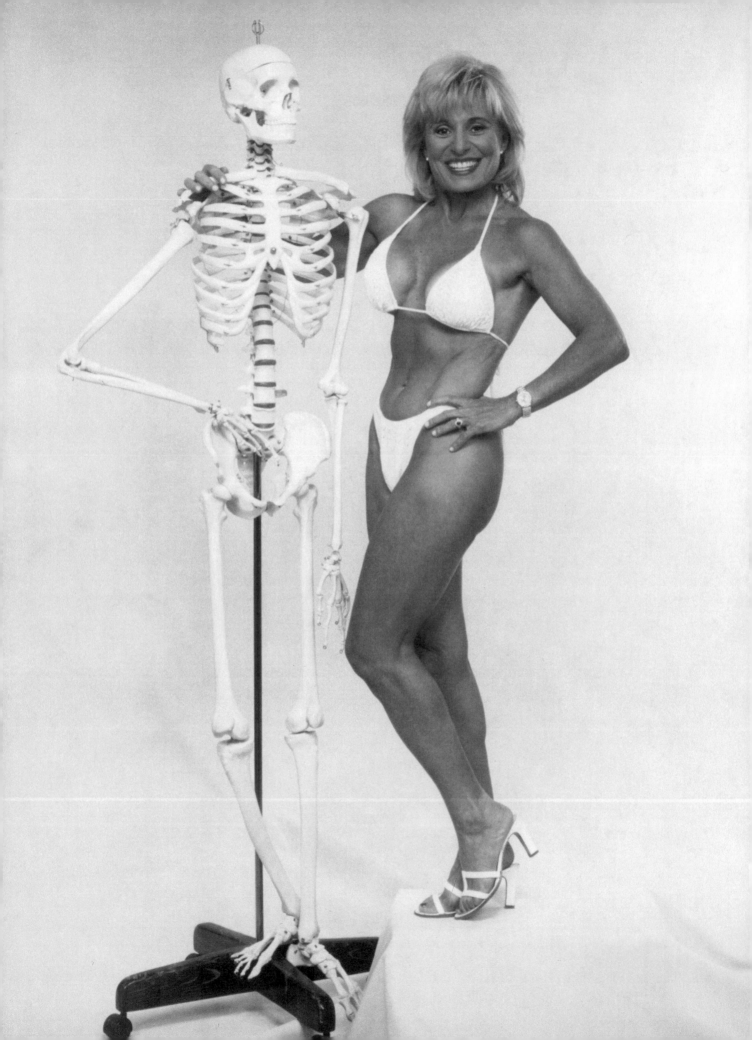

1. Build Bone, Strengthen Muscle, and Create a Beautiful Body in the Bargain

Yes, you read it right. You can build bone and strengthen, shape, and define muscle—and build an exquisite body at the same time. And you will also increase your metabolism so you can eat more without getting fat, increase your energy level, reduce your stress, and look and feel younger. You can do this by working out with light, handheld weights and following a specific routine.

Aha! Specific routine. Therein lies the secret. In order to get the promised result, you have to follow a specific plan that will exercise each and every body part to create a balanced, strong, efficient, sculpted body. This book shows you exactly how—and you can do it in just sixteen minutes a day (the standard routine) or cut your time in half, that's only eight minutes, by splitting the routine into more sessions.

How This Book Differs from My Other Exercise Books

Many of you already know me. You've seen me on the talk shows. You've used one of my previous exercise books. Maybe you've even written to me, and I've answered your questions regarding a workout in one of my books. So why buy another book? This book is different! It's the only one I've written that focuses on building bone and muscle in specific areas for strength, health, and energy. It shows you how to do this in every body part in order of importance for daily life activities, sports, and adventures—no matter what age you are. In addition, this book will give you a beautiful, shapely, toned, defined body that has no excess body fat. Your body will not only look great, but it will also feel great to the touch, and you'll have energy that you never had before.

For those of you who, like me, are already over forty or perhaps are well into your fifties, the routines in this book will not merely preserve the bone and muscle you have but, more important, will increase your bone density and replace lost muscle—and replace it with better shaped, defined, and tighter muscle than you have ever had, whether or not you are on estrogen replacement therapy. (See page 5–6 for my bone density test results without the aid of estrogen.) For those of you who are in your twenties or thirties, the routines will seem to "hold back the hand of time" and guarantee that you stay looking and feeling young and healthy well into your fifties, sixties, seventies, and older. They will serve as a hedge against osteoporosis and a host of other problems. (See chapter 2, Bone in the Bank.)

How can I promise this? I can offer medical proof. But don't take my word for it. Everything you are going to read here is being reconfirmed every day by studies done by doctors and researchers, and related in medical journals, newspapers, and books. The word is out: *Working out with light weights the right way is the fountain of youth, health, strength, and beauty.* I've been saying this for a long time, but now I have medical proof and a specific plan on how to target your most vulnerable areas—for the young, *before the problem starts;* for the middle-aged, *exactly when the problem has started;* and for the senior, *after the problem has started and has taken a toll.* It is never too late.

How Can Working Out with Weights Build Bone?

Bone is continually breaking down and being rebuilt by an automatic system in the body. But as we get older, this system slows down, and bone is not rebuilt as quickly, so we lose bone density. We now know that we can stimulate bone growth (bone density) by working out with weights, no matter what our age. If we are young, we put a rock-solid bone structure "in the bank." If we are middle-aged and don't have a solid base or even if we are elderly and have lost bone, we can build bone. Here's how it works:

Bone is made of calcium phosphate and collagen. There are hundreds of concentric rings called haversian canals within each bone. When you lift a weight, your muscles react and do work. Because muscles are attached to bones, pressure and tension are put on the bone as well. Blood flows through both the muscle and the bone, carrying nutrients to the bone-building cells. At the same time, an electrical charge shoots through the haversian canals, stimulating bone growth. This process is triggered by weight lifting.

There is a very important connection between muscle and bone strength: The more muscle you have, the denser your bones will be! Studies prove this. If you increase muscle mass, you build bone. If you reduce muscle mass, you reduce bone density. This link is so strong that archaeologists are able to calculate the muscle strength of prehistoric people by using bone strength and form as a guide. Studies show that lean body mass is the best predictor of skeletal strength.[1] So as you build bone, you are also building firm, shapely, feminine muscle.

You Can Build Bone at Any Age

In chapter 2, Bone in the Bank, I talk about building bone in your most formative "bone-peaking" years (your twenties and thirties), but here, let's talk about proof that bone can be built at *any* age.

Many studies are now being published which show that women in their forties, fifties, sixties, and all the way through their nineties can and do build bone if they work out even with light weights. The *Journal of Bone and Mineral Research* has reported a study done by Dr. L. A. Pruit and associates in which a group of seventeen women in early menopause were put on a weight-training program for nine months. Another similar group did not work out. Neither group took estrogen (hormone replacement therapy). The results were that those who worked out with weights significantly increased their lumbar bone density. Lumbar bone is the most porous bone as well as the most quickly lost; it was also the bone previously thought "impossible" to build and replace.[2]

But what if a woman is taking estrogen replacement therapy? Can she build bone that way and not work out? No. Estrogen will help preserve the bone women have, but it cannot "build" new bone. A study cited in the same journal, by Dr. M. Notelovitz and colleagues, discusses two groups of menopausal women who were given estrogen, but only one group was allowed to work out with weights. At the end of one year, the women just taking estrogen did not increase bone density, while the women taking estrogen and doing weight training significantly increased the bone density of their spine as well as their forearms.[3]

You Can Prevent and Even Reverse Osteoporosis

Weight training not only halts osteoporosis, it reverses it![4]

In her book *150 Most-Asked Questions About Osteoporosis*, Ruth Jacobowitz says, "Today, exercise physiologists believe weight lifting (resistance training) to be one of the most effective exercise regimens for osteoporosis prevention. That is because lifting weight stresses your muscles which build mass, which in turn puts stress on your bones, which can help to maintain, or even enhance, your bone density."[5]

At Fifty-four I Have the Bone Density of a Woman with Peak Bone Density—a Twenty-five to Thirty-five-year-old!

Medical experts agree that women reach their peak bone density at twenty-five to thirty-five years of age, and they lose one percent a year every year after that. But in menopause (and I was three years into it when I had the QCT-Bone

Mineral Analysis test) most women lose about 3 percent a year. If this is true, when I had the bone density test, I should have already lost about 15 to 20 percent of my bone mass. But when my bone density was measured, the result was 219.3—nearly double the bone density of an average woman my age. The doctor called me at home because he was astounded. "You went off the curve," he said. "You have the bones of a woman in her twenties." He quickly began my workout himself and recommended it to all the people in his office, especially the women.

Apparently, not only had I not lost bone mass, I had gained some—and at the time of the test, I had not taken estrogen (or hormone replacement therapy).

How Does Working Out with Weights Build Muscle?

Let's talk about muscle. You already know about the muscle-bone connection, but exactly how do muscles grow and change when you work out with weights?

When you lift more weight than usual, your muscle contracts against the resistance and calls into play muscle fibers that were formerly resting. In order to cope with the work being required of them, the muscle fibers begin to synthesize protein, and new cells are added. At the same time the muscles endure microscopic tears. The "soreness" you feel after a workout is the result of this normal microscopic tear process. When you stop working out, perhaps while you are sleeping, your muscles repair themselves. The entire process, including the "repair" during rest, causes the muscle cells to enlarge and grow stronger over time. In addition, your connecting tissues (tendons and ligaments) get stronger because they, too, are stimulated by the work being done.

Small Shapely Muscles—Not the "Bodybuilder" Kind!

I almost skipped this section! Why? Today, most women know that you don't just pick up a weight and wake up looking like Arnold. But just in case you're worried, I want to assure you that by working out with light weights for such a short amount of time, there is no way you could possibly build huge, hulking muscles. In fact, female bodybuilders wish it were that easy. They use hundred-pound weights and more, and work out for hours a day. You, on the other hand, will work out only eight to sixteen minutes a day (thirty-two at the most if you go the extra mile) and lift only one, two, and three pounds to start (fifteen to twenty pounds much later if you choose).

Where do we get the idea that we will bulk up if we use weights? We see female bodybuilders on TV who quite often look like men with women's heads attached. Well, chances are that the ones who really look like men, in addition to working out with heavy weights for hours a day, ingest steroids—male hormones called testosterone, a substance that women also produce naturally in a very small quantity. When women take this hormone in great quantities, their muscle-making ability multiplies, but in addition to getting huge muscles, many of them develop other male traits, such as facial hair, deepened voices, and rougher skin.

So don't worry about looking like a man. You'll be using very light weights. And you certainly won't be taking steroids.

You Can Reverse the Aging Process at Any Age

I've always said that women who work out with weights look and feel and indeed are physically ten years younger than their chronological age. Why? They replace lost muscle and bone, improve their posture, increase their energy levels, and walk with the same spring in their step that they had ten years before. But recently, to my joy, I've been proven wrong: Their bodies are, in fact, fifteen to twenty years younger. Yes. Miriam E. Nelson, Ph.D., who is the associate chief of the Human Physiology Laboratory at the Jean Mayer USDA Human Nutrition Research Center on Aging at Tufts University, and professor at the School of Nutrition Science and Policy, studied forty postmenopausal women, none of whom was on hormone replacement therapy. She divided the group in two. Twenty of the women lifted weights twice a week, and the other group did not. The group that did nothing lost bone and muscle mass. The group that worked out with weights were "fifteen to twenty years more youthful."[6]

But what about older people? In 1991, *The New York Times Magazine* presented a study done at Tufts University. William Evans, the director of the physiology laboratory at the Human Nutrition Research Center on Aging, took women and men ranging in age from eighty-seven to ninety-six and put them on an eight-week weight-training program. The average strength increase in the front thigh muscles for the group of nine was almost 200 percent![7]

Raise Your Metabolism by 15 Percent in Twelve Weeks and Eat More Without Getting Fat

It has been medically established that our metabolism drops by 2 percent every ten years, and doctors are saying today that this drop starts at the age of twenty! By the age of thirty we lose approximately half a pound of muscle a year. And for every ounce of muscle we lose, our body not only becomes "flabbier" but our metabolism goes down because muscle is the only body material that is active twenty-four hours a day.

What does this mean? By the time you are fifty, your metabolism has dropped by at least 10 to 15 percent. But it gets worse. Once a woman hits menopause and stops menstruating, she no longer burns the 20,000 calories a year that is burned by the "period" itself (the loss of blood). Since it takes 3,000 excess calories to produce a pound of body fat, most women gain 6.5 to 7 pounds in the year or two after menopause even if their diet and activity have not changed at all.

Don't get depressed! I have an immediate and foolproof remedy to tune up your metabolism to compensate for the slowing metabolism, and you can tune it up higher than it ever was, as I did, so you can eat plenty before you start gaining weight. After doing this workout for only twelve weeks, you can raise your metabolism by 15 percent so that you can eat 15 percent more than you used to eat without getting fat![8] And when you tune up your metabolism even higher, you put more muscle on your body over time—as I did.

How does muscle tune up your metabolism? Every pound of muscle you add to your body burns about 40 to 50 extra calories a day. You'll lose pounds of fat while gaining the muscle. So if you're overweight, you will lose weight on the scale, but the more dramatic change will be in your size. Muscle weighs more than fat, but it takes up less space. Think of muscle as a silver dollar, and fat as a kitchen sponge. The silver dollar weighs more, but the kitchen sponge takes up more space. The analogy holds true even to how it feels. Put your hand on a soft, fatty thigh and then on a muscular thigh. Which feels spongy and which feels hard?

One more point. I weigh 115 pounds, and I'm five feet tall. I wear a size 4 dress, but before I worked out, I wore a size 10 at the same weight and looked chunky. If I stand next to another woman my height and weight who never worked out, she will look heavy and wear about three sizes larger than I do. This is because I'm made of dense muscle that takes up less space and burns fat twenty-four hours a day. She is made of spongy fat that is lighter in weight and takes up more space. So once you do the workout, you'll see a major change in the mirror and in clothing size, but not necessarily on the scale.

Improve Your Strength, Balance, and Sports Ability

When you work out with weights (also called "strength training"), you improve your strength and become more capable when playing any sport. By following the workout in this book, your shoulders, back, arms, and legs will be stronger so you can better swing that tennis or racquetball racket, or that golf club. Your back, knees, and arms will be more powerful so you can ski with more stamina. Your legs and total body musculature will be stronger so that you can increase your endurance for running and walking. And, yes, if you do the optional weight-bearing aerobic additions, you will also improve your cardiovascular ability! Chapter 4 gives specific workouts for your sport.

We've talked about strength, but what about balance? We need it for everything from getting out of bed in the morning to walking—not to mention sports activities. Believe it or not, balance starts to decline as early as our forties. Small wonder that many elderly people fall so often. But this doesn't have to happen.

Studies show that working out with weights improves balance. One researcher reported that after breaking her hip, a seventy-year-old woman began working out with weights as part of her recovery program. This woman now cross-country skis with her grandchildren, and hikes with them as well. In fact, she has been seen shoveling snow off the roof of her house, having climbed there with no problem at all![9]

Reduce Your Stress Level

We've always known that doing aerobic workouts helps reduce stress by providing a natural high as a result of "endorphins," but now we know that working out with weights does the same—and more. A study done at Tufts University revealed that weight training was able to take the place of mild antidepressants for a group of women. My own twenty-five-year-old daughter, Marthe, is testimony to this. Whenever she is under stress, she does a weight workout. She says, "No matter how stressed out I am, after working out with weights, I feel as if a burden has been lifted. I feel so relaxed. It's really amazing—like medicine."

Do the Weight-Bearing Aerobics and Get a Triple Whammy

In addition to the weight workout (strength training), you will have the option of doing weight-bearing aerobics, an option I strongly advise. Weight-bearing aerobics deliver a triple-whammy bonus when it comes to fitness. You get your heart and lungs in shape and at the same time burn off excess body fat. And in the bargain, you increase bone density.

If this is so, why not simply do weight-bearing aerobic exercises and forget training with weights? Because working out with weights increases bone density over every single body part. You are in full control of each bone you thicken and the muscle you build and shape. Aerobics is a more general workout for the back, legs, or spine. In addition, working out with weights gives you a greater increase in bone density than weight-bearing aerobics. Finally—and to me this is a key point—there is no other way to sculpt, define, tighten, and tone each and every muscle to give the proper shape to every body part: arms, buttocks, hips, thighs, stomach. You must use weights—and in a very specific way.

What are weight-bearing exercises? Well, for starters, swimming is not a weight-bearing exercise. When you swim, the water, not your body, "bears" the weight. Weight-bearing aerobic exercises are jogging, running, walking on the ground or on a treadmill, climbing stairs (stair-stepping and stair-climbing machines are not quite as weight-bearing as climbing real stairs), skiing (downhill or cross-country), jumping rope, and dancing, both social and low-impact aerobic.

In addition to swimming, the other aerobic exercises that are not weight-bearing are workouts on exercise and functional bicycles, and water aerobics. Yes, there is a slight element of "weight-bearing" in these, but not a whole lot. (See chapter 9, Bone-Building Aerobics, for more details, and chapter 4, Creative Workouts, for ways to incorporate these into your weight-training routine.)

What About Diet and Hormone Replacement Therapy?

Calcium, vitamin D, and a host of other nutrients are essential for bone and muscle health. But how do you obtain all these food elements and still lose excess body fat (if you are overweight)? A whole chapter is devoted to this (see chapter 10), but in the meantime, rest assured that you will be able to eat delicious, nutritious food without feeling starved and without using diet pills of any kind.

Every woman must decide for herself whether or not to go on hormone replacement therapy (HRT), which is a combination of estrogen and progesterone. There is no doubt that estrogen replacement once menopause begins prevents rapid bone deterioration (and helps with a host of other problems, too), but it does not "build" bone. Whether or not you go on HRT, you need this workout.

Health and Beauty, Too

Okay, so you're just doing this workout for your health. Well, whether you like it or not, you're going to have a sexier, more beautifully shaped, tight, toned body, so you'd better cover it up or expect trouble.

I used to work out for the "beauty" aspect alone. Once I turned fifty, though, I began to see all the health problems that couch potatoes had and thanked God that I had inadvertently been doing the best health-strength-longevity routine. I decided to perfect it and make it ideal for bone and muscle health while keeping the beauty aspects because as you get older, if you don't have your health, very soon you won't have your life—at least not a life worth living. Hence this book.

Do the Workout at Home with Inexpensive Handheld Weights

The good news is that you can do the workout at home with handheld weights called "dumbbells," and you can purchase these weights at fifty cents a pound by looking under "exercise equipment" in the yellow pages. (In chapter 4 you'll learn exactly what to buy.) You don't need to spend more than about $10.00, tax included, to get started. Of course, if you want to get the fancy colored weights, you may spend a lot more. And indeed, as you get stronger, you will be buying heavier weights—but even at your strongest, you won't be investing hundreds of dollars.

But what if you want to use exercise machines, either at home or at a fitness center? You will find that, except when there is no possible substitute, there is a "machines" section for every exercise. I like the dumbbells better, but once in a while, for variety, I'll go to a gym and use the machines, too.

You Can Do This Workout at Any Age and at Any Weight

Whether you're sixteen or sixty, seventeen or seventy, eighteen or eighty, and whether you're overweight or exactly the right weight, you can do this workout. (If you are the right weight, you may need muscle tone, and for sure you can use the bone-building aspect. If you're overweight, you'll lose your excess body fat and get to that toned body you've always wanted.) In short, with your doctor's approval, you can get started right away and enjoy the wonderful benefits of weight training, the fountain of youth. What about men? Yes, men can do it, too!

Choose a Workout: Eight, Sixteen, or Thirty-two Minutes

This part will thrill you. You can work out only eight minutes a day and still get the promised results. If you choose the eight-minute workout, you will be doing something different each day—working one-fourth of your body each day. You will then repeat the cycle. You can have a day off or, better, just keep going and not take any days off. You can do this because you're never working the same body parts two days in a row. (More about this in chapters 3 and 4.)

If you are more ambitious and want to do the regular workout, you will work out sixteen minutes a day. You'll do half of your body on your first workout day and the other half on your second workout day. You will then repeat the cycle. You can keep repeating the cycle or take a day off after having repeated the cycle two or three times. (More about this in chapter 4.)

For those of you who want to have more days off and are ambitious, you can do your entire body in one workout day. Then you *must* take a day off. (You can even take two days off.) Then you repeat the entire body exercises during the same week. If you do your entire body twice in a week, you will be getting the same workout as if you did the sixteen-minute workout four days a week. (More about this in chapter 4.)

Doing the Max

There is no reason to do more than the above. But I know you! You'll probably say, "Hey, I love this. Can't I do more?" Well, you can do the ultra max. You can work your entire body three days a week for thirty-two minutes just as long as you take a day off after each weight workout. This is the maximum. When I say "a day off," I mean a day off the weights. You can still opt to do your "weight-bearing aerobics" on any day—whether you are weight training or taking a day off. (More on this in chapter 4.)

What You Will Get from This Workout

Increased strength—stronger muscles

Increased bone density—stronger bones

Toned, defined, firm, shapely body

Reduced dress or pant size in approximately three weeks

Increased metabolism so you burn more fat twenty-four hours a day

Loss of excess body fat, replaced with tight, toned muscles in twelve weeks

Improved stamina: sports, life tasks, and you know what else (begins with s)

Improved balance and agility

Improved posture

Increased energy

Improved outlook on life, self-image, and self-confidence

Reduced stress level

Reduced pain from arthritis

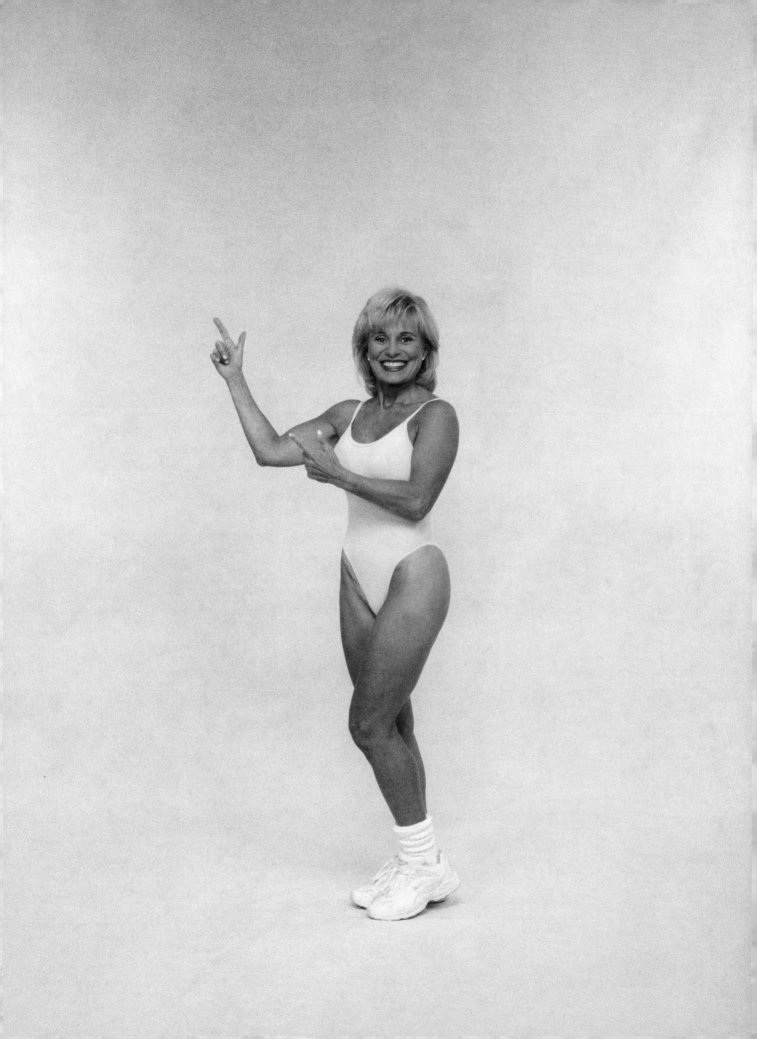

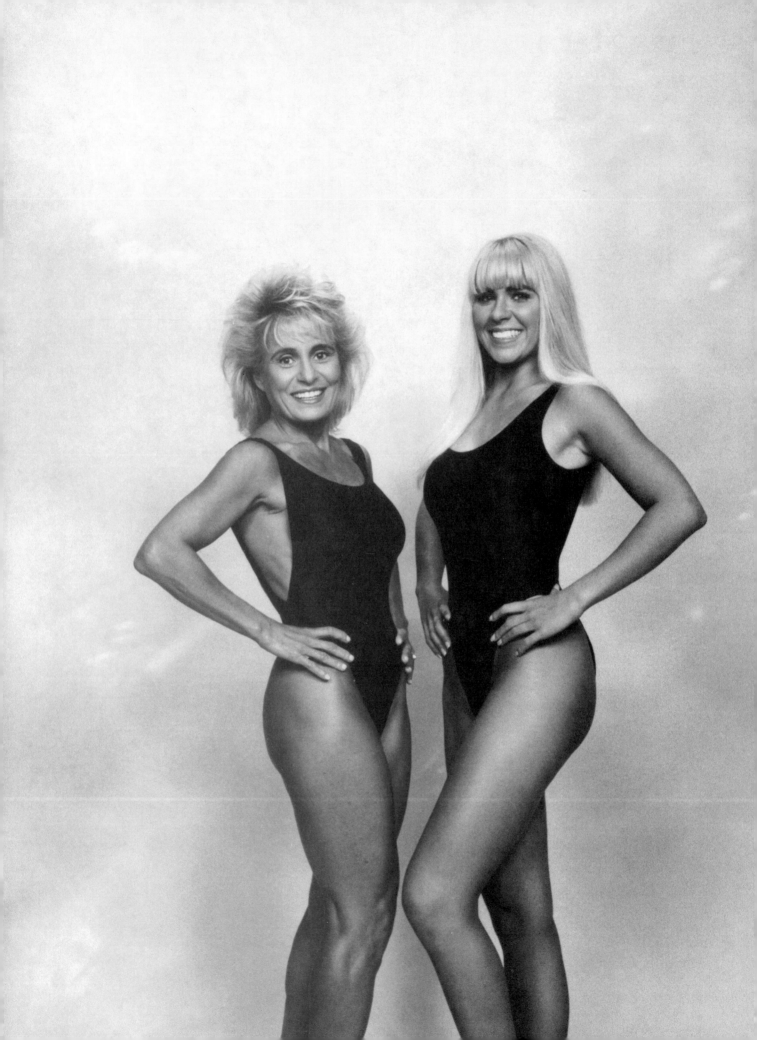

2. Bone in the Bank

Wouldn't it be wonderful if we could build and develop such a strong bone base as we age that we would never, ever be in danger of osteoporosis and, in the bargain, create a beautiful, tight, toned body? What if, along with all this, we could make ourselves so strong and agile that we could perform any task or sport with the greatest of ease?

Well, we can, and we can do it at any age. No matter how old you are, it's not too early or late to put "bone in the bank." My daughter Marthe, featured with me in the photograph, started working out with weights on a regular basis at the age of eighteen. She had gone to college, gained weight, and realized weight training was the only way to lose weight and keep it off without starving and at the same time tone, define, and improve her shape. What Marthe didn't realize was that she was building bone in her peak bone-building years while she was building muscle.

At twenty-five, Marthe is still working out, and she tells me that it not only allows her to eat more without getting fat, but it is also her remedy for stress. "I could start out in the worst mood, but five minutes into the workout I seem to forget my problems. And by the time I'm finished, I always feel better. Not sometimes but always. You can bet on it. I think people wouldn't need to go on antidepressants if they worked out on a regular basis."

Bone Building from Twenty to Thirty-five for Optimum Peak

Most experts believe that bone density reaches its natural peak between thirty and thirty-five. In order to ensure that you get your maximum bone base—that bone in the bank—it's a good idea to work out with weights. We can now prove that working out with weights increases bone density in young women and solidifies the lifetime bone base. This is not to say that bone cannot be built in later years. Of course it can, and it is indeed one of the purposes of this book!

To cite only one of many studies, a group of active women in their twenties and thirties were divided into two groups: One group did only aerobics workouts, with no weights. The other group worked out with weights. Both groups were tested for bone density before and after the six-month experiment. The women

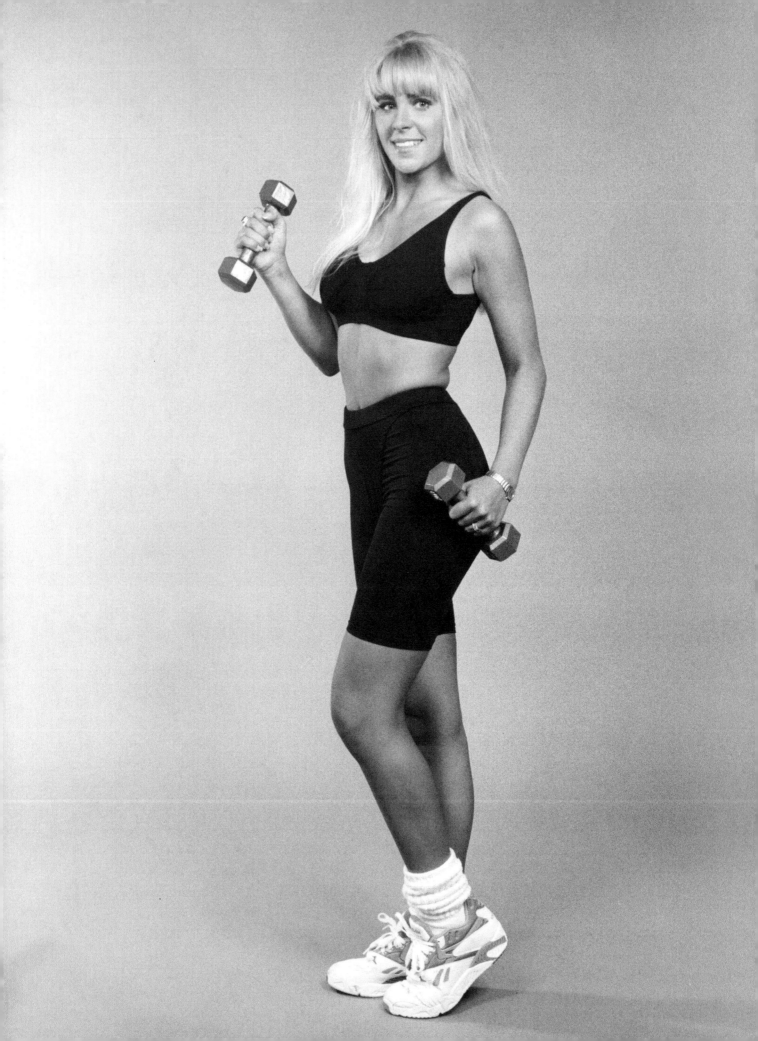

who worked out with weights had increased their bone density significantly, while the women who did the aerobic workouts alone increased their bone density by only a fraction.[1]

But what part does diet play in the building of bone density in the peak years? While it is true that eating a proper amount of calcium-rich foods (or at least taking calcium supplements) cannot *build* bone, a deficiency of this mineral can *hinder the body from developing its peak bone mass*.[2] I'll talk more about calcium in chapter 10, but in the meantime, remember that to ensure you reach your optimum bone peak during your natural bone-building years, you should have enough calcium on a daily basis.

How Is Bone Naturally Built in the Body?

There is a bone-building and bone-renewing process taking place in your body all the time. As mentioned before, bone is continually tearing down and healing itself. Here's how it works: "Osteoclasts" (bone-breakdown cells) destroy old, damaged bone. This damaged bone is reabsorbed into the blood. At the same time, "osteoblasts" (bone-building cells) replace the damaged bone with new bone by producing the protein collagen and calcifying that collagen. This bone breakdown and renewal is called "bone remodeling." When the bone-remodeling system breaks down—when more old bone is destroyed than new bone is made—the result is thinning bones and, possibly, osteoporosis.

The only way to ensure that the system does not break down is to work out with weights and, if possible, do weight-bearing exercises as well. And, of course, a proper amount of calcium-rich foods or calcium supplements should be consumed.

There Are Two Types of Bone

The bone-building process is taking place for two types of bone in your body: "trabecular" and "cortical." Trabecular bone is the softer, spongy, more loosely packed bone, such as the backbone, ribs, and breastbone. However, some trabecular material is found in the inner section of almost every bone. Cortical bone, on the other hand, is harder and denser. The arm and leg bones are made mostly of cortical bone. In addition, this hard material is found in small amounts on the surface of nearly every bone in the body.

Surprise: Bone Loss Occurs Well Before Menopause

Many women allow themselves to be falsely comforted by the thought that it is only after menopause (around the age of fifty) that bone loss begins to occur.

Studies show, however, that half of the total backbone loss occurs before, not after, menopause.[3] Why does this loss occur? Lack of exercise is the main culprit, along with improper diet. But there is no reason for this to happen to you. By investing a minimum of eight to sixteen minutes a day, you can ensure that the opposite will happen: You'll have "sexy bones," so to speak, because they will be covered by the shapely muscles that develop while making them.

Bank Robbery: Catch the Thief!

When a woman reaches menopause, lack of estrogen can cause bone loss. But young people who still have plenty of estrogen can also lose bone—not because of lack of estrogen but because they are unaware of the invasion of bone thieves in their lives. We've already discussed lack of exercise and poor nutrition, but after those thieves come cigarette smoking and the consumption of too much alcohol.

Excessive caffeine can also leech the bones of calcium, and extremely high protein diets can, too. Diets very high in sodium are not good, either. Finally, starvation diets and excessive exercise to the point where menstruation stops and estrogen production is drastically reduced can cause problems. Interestingly, most young women don't have the problem of exercising too much. They exercise too little. (Of course, older women are equally affected by these bone thieves.)

True or False: Debunking Some Myths About Building Muscle and Bone

As discussed in chapter 1, the building of bone and the building of muscle go hand in hand. The stronger your muscle, the stronger your bone. The more muscle you build, the more bone you build. But before you start building bone and muscle, and putting them into your health bank, I'd like to put your mind at ease and debunk some myths about working out. In addition, I'd like to help you form realistic expectations from your workout.

1. There is no such thing as a "fountain of youth" exercise.
   False. I've said it for years in all my weight-training books, and the medical experts are finally catching up with me. Working out with weights literally reverses the aging process. It restores and builds new muscle and bone; it restores and gives new strength and energy; it reshapes, tightens, and tones the body; and it makes you look and feel ten to twenty years younger. It even improves your sex life—and motivates you to have one if you don't. (In fact, it could get you in trouble. Watch out!)

2. **Young women don't have to exercise!**

> *False.* You should exercise while you're young in order to build peak bone mass before you start to lose that 1 percent a year beginning around age thirty-five. Of course, if you are older, no problem. You can work out and regain what you lost so far, and more. (See page 24. Some doctors believe bone begins to erode even earlier—and at a faster pace.)

3. **Lifting weights is fine for young people, but after a certain age, it's impossible to regain lost bone, much less build new bone.**

> *False.* Not only can you regain lost bone at any age, but you can gain new bone even into your eighties and older. Study after study proves this. Everyone should check with her doctor, of course, before starting any exercise program.

4. **Any exercise is better than no exercise.**

> *True.* Rather than stagnate, it's better to exercise. But in reality, any exercise where you are standing as opposed to sitting is likely to build bone. Multiple studies show that sedentary people of every age have much lower bone density than active people of every age. People who are bedridden have been found to lose as much as 1 percent of their lumbar spine mass in only a week! To regain bone loss, exercises done sitting in bed do no good, but just standing for two hours regains bone loss caused by a week of bed rest.[4]

5. **Exercise helps prevent breast cancer.**

> *True.* Believe it or not, we are now finding proof that an active life can help prevent breast cancer. In fact, a *New York Times* article reports that just 3.8 hours a week of exercise (this can include your bone-building workout plus your extra bone-building aerobics) reduces the risk of cancer by 50 percent.
>
> The study was done by Dr. Leslie Bernstein of the University of Southern California School of Medicine in Los Angeles. In a group of one thousand women, it was discovered that those who exercised 3.8 hours or more a week were less than half as likely to develop breast cancer as inactive women.[5]

6. **Exercise machines are very high-tech and give you a better workout than the old-fashioned handheld "dumbbells."**

> *False.* Even today, with all the fancy air-pressure and other machines, handheld dumbbells are your best bet overall. Why? You completely control the weights, and you are forced to do all the work (no cheating). Handheld weights are inexpensive and portable. With one simple set of dumbbells you can exercise all nine body parts and, in the bargain, do five or more different exercises for each of those body parts. Machines, on the other hand, allow you to exercise only a few body parts, with a few exercises each. And if you have one of those home gym

machines, more often than not you waste so much time adjusting the apparatus for various exercises that you lose a lot of the efficacy of the workout.

Are machines worthless? Of course not. If you have a machine at home or wish to go to a fitness center, you will find machine substitutes in this book for almost every exercise. (When you don't find one, it's because, to my knowledge, it doesn't exist.)

7. Once you start working out with weights, you'd better never stop, or the muscle will turn to fat and your bones will disintegrate!

False. Muscle and fat cells are completely different, both structurally and functionally. When you build muscles, as discussed on page 8, you actually lose fat because you increase your metabolism. But what happens if you stop working out? Your muscles eventually revert to their original condition, but it takes as long as your cumulative workout time to do this. For example, if you worked out for a year, it would take a year for you to lose the muscle tone you had gained. But if you ever start working out again, it takes only one-third the time to get back that muscle. So, in a way, working out with weights is muscle in the bank. The same may apply to bones.

8. You'd better not work out with weights if you're overweight. You'll only get muscles and look bigger than you already look.

False. In fact, muscles take up less space than fat and help to burn fat. If you work out, chances are you'll go down a dress or pant size before you even see a change on the scale. In addition, if you wait until you've lost the weight to start working out, you'll be flabby, and your bones will not get the benefit of the weight-training workout. Why put it off? If you work out while following a sensible healthy diet, instead of feeling punished and deprived of food, you'll think like an athlete: "I'm in training. I'm eating for my strength, energy, and health."

9. If you hear popping or grinding noises as you work out, it means you are too old to work out.

False. Medical experts say that when you hear a popping sound, it means your ligaments and tendons are changing position! In other words, when you move your body part, your connective tissue repositions itself over your moving joints. Interestingly, I've heard this popping for years, but only for the first few repetitions of certain exercises. Medical experts say this is exactly when you should hear it.

Grinding comes from the rubbing of the cartilage at the ends of the bones against each other—and is most prevalent when you've had a previous injury in the area. Again, no problem—unless there is pain. In any case, to be sure of your personal situation, I advise that you check with your doctor before continuing the workout so you can enjoy yourself without fear.

10. You must exercise the entire body in order to get results! You can't spot-reduce or spot-change.

False. You can and do change and reshape each body part as you exercise that body part individually, although other body parts are often partially affected at the same time. For example, when you exercise your arms, they receive the main benefit of the workout. Your leg bones and muscles do not become stronger, nor do your hip or buttocks bones and muscles. But your shoulders and chest benefit slightly.

You can shape muscle and build bone density just on your arms! You can do the same for just your legs, for just your back, and so on. But why do that? It's much better for your looks (total body symmetry) and health (total body balance) to exercise your entire body.

Where did we get the idea that we can't change one body part at a time? From the fact that you can't spot-reduce by dieting. When you diet, your body loses fat from its favorite storage areas and also from its entire structure. For example, if you're thirty pounds overweight and you go on a low-fat calorie-restricted eating plan, in time you'll lose thirty pounds. The bulk of that weight will probably be lost from your stomach, hips, butt, and thighs because that's where most of it was stored. But some of it will also come off your chest, shoulders, back, face, neck, and so on.

The only way to spot-change and build is by working out with weights the right way—as described in this and other books (see bibliography).

11. Muscle soreness means you are probably injured.

False. Muscle soreness is a perfectly normal result of working out, and it happens because of microscopic tears in your muscle fibers, ligaments, and tendons. The slight temporary internal swelling causes this soreness. If you are sore, you should rejoice. Why? As previously mentioned, this same tearing down process eventually causes the muscle to become denser, stronger, firmer, and, with this workout, reshaped into a more appealing form.

When you have an injury, you will probably know it because there will be a sharp and/or continual pain as you try to work out. But if you're in any doubt whatsoever, check with your doctor. The most common weight-training injuries occur when the tendons become inflamed (tendinitis) or ligaments are torn or the covering (fascia) of the muscle itself is torn (fasciitis).

It is very unlikely that you will ever have such an injury with this workout because you will be lifting very light handheld weights in a controlled manner. When you do increase your weights, you will do so gradually, as instructed in chapter 4.

12. If you feel sore, you should stop working out until the soreness goes away.

False. The ideal thing to do is to work out anyway. You'll probably forget about the soreness after a few minutes of working out because the sore muscles feel "massaged" by the circulating blood and feel less stiff. After a few weeks, you won't feel any more soreness—unless, of course, you work out extra hard one day or try some new exercises. What would happen if you stopped working out until the soreness went away? You guessed it: You'd be on an endless sore cycle because you would be always starting anew. I say bite the bullet! Work through the soreness. Enjoy it. And in your mind, draw a circle around every sore part because the muscles and bones in that area are being made stronger and tighter.

But what if you feel no soreness after your first few workouts? Be sure you are not cheating. Are you making complete movements, full repetitions? Are you doing all of the sets, all of the exercises, or are you leaving some out? Are you keeping up a decent pace? Are you resting too long between sets? Are your weights too light? If none of the above is true and you don't feel sore, don't worry. Everyone's body is not the same. Just be grateful that you are one of the lucky ones who isn't discomforted much when the muscles are "tearing down and being rebuilt." Your body may just ignore this process!

13. If the workout takes longer or shorter than the time the book says, you're doing it wrong.

False. After your break-in period, you may just move faster or slower than the "average" person. Don't worry about it. Try to keep it moving and don't rush it, but no matter what you do, your pace may be different from other people. I go faster than the time allowed in the book and usually finish the sixteen-minute workout in nine or ten minutes, and so do many other people. But there are also many people who go slower and take up to twenty minutes. If you're taking much longer, you really should pick up your pace.

14. Men don't need this workout. It's only for women.

False. Men need this workout, too, for muscles as well as bones. Men do not suffer as quickly and as severely as women do from osteoporosis. (Their problems become severe in their seventies, while women have to worry as early as their fifties.) The reason is that men naturally produce the muscle-making bone-enhancing hormone testosterone in much greater quantities than women do and therefore start out with about 30 percent more bone mass in the first place. In addition, while the bone-enhancing female hormone estrogen diminishes as early as the late forties in women, the bone-enhancing male hormone testosterone is sustained at nearly the same level throughout a man's lifetime.

By the age of seventy, most men lose about one-seventh of their bone mass, and in their older years, one out of eight men will suffer a bone fracture.

But men should work out with weights for yet another reason, and in my opinion this is the most important one of all: to prevent and reverse muscle atrophy! A man's muscles atrophy by about half a pound every year after thirty. And by the time he's forty-five, his whole body shape will have changed for the worse even if he weighs not a pound more. I am reminded of the many men who brag, "I weigh the same as I did in college." But what's wrong with this picture? Skinny, sloping shoulders, toothpick arms, a little paunch, a narrow back, "love handles," and so on. Who is kidding whom? If a man wants to look good and feel firm, he had better lift those weights.

15. If you do the minimum bone-building workout of only eight minutes a day, you're fooling yourself.

False. The eight-minute workout exercises your entire body once every four days—nearly twice a week. What's more, even the eight-minute workout has nearly triple the amount of exercise that you get in many other workout books written by medical doctors and researchers. And these books with minimal workouts even promise increased muscle and bone! You can therefore imagine what you'll get from this workout—even in eight minutes. Of course, if you want to increase your benefits still more, do the regular sixteen-minute workout.

16. Thinning bone can be made denser by eating a calcium-rich diet or taking calcium supplements.

False. While it is true that 98 percent of the calcium found in our bodies is located in the bones and that a calcium-deficient diet will result in our bones never reaching their peak capacity and thinning faster than they should, *calcium cannot build or restore porous bone.* You must be active and, at best, work out with weights and do weight-bearing exercises to restore and increase bone density.[6]

17. If you're badly out of shape or have thinning bones, you dare not work with weights.

False. If you consult with your doctor and use the easy-does-it break-in plan, you can work out with weights at any age—even in your nineties—no matter how badly out of shape you are. In fact, the more badly out of shape you are, the more you need this program. But don't rush it. Take your time. You'll be amazed how strong you'll become if you gently coax yourself as you go along. One-pound weights may seem like a ton now, but in two weeks they'll feel like feathers, and so on. In a year you'll think you are an amazon. I can't wait until you write and tell me about it.

18. You dare not work out with weights if you have arthritis.

False. In fact, there is some proof that working out with weights actually helps reduce pain from arthritis and improves the range of motion, in addition to increasing muscle strength and improving the shape and tone of the muscle.[7] I've received letters from women who, after using my workout with their doctor's permission to reduce pain from arthritis, improved bone density at the same time.

19. Working out with weights can do nothing for your heart and lungs. Only aerobic activities can do that.

False. While it is true that aerobic activities are the best for increasing heart and lung capacity and endurance, working out with weights improves the muscle-to-fat ratio of your body and, in that sense, helps your heart. In addition, when you put more muscle on your body, you increase your metabolism so that you burn even more fat. And working out with weights can increase your good cholesterol (high-density lipoprotein, or HDL). Finally, weight training helps to increase your aerobic endurance ability so you can also get the well-known aerobic heart-lung effect mentioned above.

20. The only people who need to worry about thinning bones are older women.

False. While most doctors agree that women begin to lose up to 1 percent of bone each year after age thirty-five, some doctors believe that bone mass begins to erode at the rate of 2 percent each year as early as thirty. The National Osteoporosis Foundation points out that while it is true postmenopausal women and, for that matter, everyone over sixty-five are at the greatest risk, women of any age are at risk if they have temporarily lost their periods (perhaps due to undereating); have a family history of osteoporosis; have broken a bone; have small body frames; have too little calcium in their diet; smoke, drink, or use caffeine excessively; take the following medications: aluminum antacids, barbiturate anticonvulsants, cholestyramine, cortisone, cyclosporin A, gloccocorticoid steroids, heparin, hydrocortisone, loop diuretics, methotrexate, phenytoin, prednisone, and thyroxine; or have had the following treatments: chemotherapy, gastrectomy, hysterectomy, oophorectomy, or organ transplants.

Other medical authorities add these risk factors to the list: being Asian or Caucasian; small-boned or thin women who don't exercise; and those who experience early menopause or imbibe more than two carbonated drinks a day.

21. Weight training cannot improve balance; in fact, it makes you clumsy because it builds muscle.

False. We now have studies that prove weight training greatly improves balance. As muscle strength increases, balance improves. One study showed a 14 percent improvement in balance after one year of very moderate strength training.[8]

22. People who are lactose intolerant are doomed to bad bones since they can't drink milk or consume dairy products without getting sick.

False. Lactose intolerance is caused by the body's inability to break down the sugar "lactose" into a digestible form. Statistics show that 30 million Americans have some form of this problem.

Since lactose is found in all dairy products, those who have this problem used to be doomed, but today caplets can be taken before consuming a dairy product that resolve the whole issue. There are also dairy products especially made for the lactose intolerant, such as brands of milk and cottage cheese. In any case, you can get calcium from the other high-calcium food items listed on page 169 and take a calcium supplement.

3. Preparing for the Workout

Now that you know why this workout will deliver a world of benefits no matter what age you are, it's time to learn some simple workout terms that will be used in the exercise instructions. It's also important for you to know some specific information on muscles and muscle movement, and where muscle and bone is located in your body. As you work out, I want you to picture your muscles and bones being stimulated by your movements so you can cooperate with this growth and shaping process. I want you to focus on your working bone and muscles, and "tell" them to grow and develop into their ideal form. It's a good idea to refer to the muscle-bone diagrams and descriptions before you do a workout until you have a clear picture in your mind of the muscles and bones that are being targeted by the particular exercises you are doing. Some experts believe that such focusing increases the efficacy of the workout by as much as 50 percent.

Exercise Terms

Breathing Naturally: to inhale and exhale in an instinctive, as opposed to conscious, manner. You will often be reminded in the exercise instructions to breathe naturally. Some experts feel that you should breathe out (exhale) on the flex part of the exercise and breathe in (inhale) on the stretch part of the exercise. This would be necessary if you were lifting very heavy weights and needed to use every bit of energy for each "thrust" of the weights. You are not involved in such lifting!

Continual Pressure: the willful flexing of the muscle throughout the exercise—including applying tension on the stretch part of the movement. (When pressure is applied to the stretch part, it's called "dynamic tension.")

Exercise: a specific movement for a particular muscle, designed to strengthen and reshape the muscle and increase the density of the bone. For example, the palms-up wrist curl is an exercise designed to strengthen, define, and sculpt the muscles in the forearm and to strengthen and thicken the wrist bones.

Flex: the shortening of the muscle fibers when squeezed together. For example, your biceps muscle is flexed when you bend your arm, but you can "flex" that same muscle even more by tightening it yourself. You can do this by imagining a doctor coming at your biceps with a long needle. You would "flex" to protect that muscle. Another way to imagine flexing is to picture someone about to punch you in the stomach. You "flex" your stomach—you harden it to protect it. In the exercise instructions I will continually say "flex" your muscles.

Giant Set: performing three or more exercises without taking a rest. You can giant-set by doing your first set of each exercise for a given body part before you take a rest, then doing your second set for each exercise for that body part before taking another rest, then finally doing your third set for each exercise in that body part. You could make the giant set even more intense by not taking the rests. In this case, you would be "speed-giant-setting." After you get very comfortable with this workout, perhaps in a few months, you could giant-set if you wish to do so.

Pyramid System: adding weight to each set at the expense of a few repetitions. The pyramid system for your beginning weights will look like this:

SET 1: 12 repetitions with 1 pound
SET 2: 10 repetitions with 2 pounds
SET 3: 8 repetitions with 3 pounds

Technically speaking, the above is the "modified" pyramid system. The true pyramid adds two more sets, for a total of ten. For the purposes of this workout, the modified pyramid system is most effective.

Repetition, or "Rep": one complete movement of an exercise, from start to finish. For example, one repetition of the palms-up wrist curl is the raising of the wrists upward (holding a dumbbell in the hand) to the highest point and then lowering the wrist downward to the lowest point. See page 119 for a photograph illustrating this exercise.

Rest: a pause between sets or exercises. The reason for resting is to give the working muscle time to recover so that it can deal with the next set of exercises. If your goal were to get huge muscles, you would have to use very heavy weights and rest as long as a minute after each set. Fortunately, since your goal is to get smaller sculpted muscles along with increased bone density, you will be using lighter weights and rest only fifteen seconds between sets. Later, when you become familiar with the exercises, you will find yourself shortening or even eliminating the rests.

Set: a given number of repetitions of a specific exercise that are performed without a rest. In this workout you will perform twelve repetitions for your *first* set of most exercises, ten repetitions for your second set, and eight repetitions for your third set.

Speed-Set: when you don't take a rest after a set but simply proceed to the next set and then the next, and so on. I love to speed-set. You can, too, but wait until you are really comfortable with the workout.

Stretch: the elongation of the muscle fibers. Using the above example, when you elongate your arm, your biceps muscle is "stretched." But you can add to that stretch by allowing yourself to feel it and flow with it, letting those muscle fibers elongate to the maximum. Interestingly, recent research shows that it is on the "stretch" or lengthening part of the weight-lifting exercise that the muscle is most strengthened, so don't rush that part. I will continually remind you of this in the exercise instructions.

Workout Expressions

The following are definitions of general workout terms.

Aerobic Exercise: a physical fitness activity, using the larger muscles of the body, that causes the pulse to reach a rate of 60 to 80 percent of its capacity and stay that way for twelve minutes or longer, supported by the body's natural flow of oxygen. (Some authorities insist that in order to achieve an "aerobic effect" one must work for twenty minutes uninterrupted; however, more and more exercise specialists are beginning to agree that one can achieve an aerobic effect in even ten minutes.)

To figure out your maximum pulse rate, subtract your age from 220 and multiply the result by 60 percent for the minimum aerobic effect. For a higher aerobic effect, multiply it by 70 to 80 percent.

Anaerobic Exercise: a physical fitness activity that is too strenuous to be supported by the body's natural flow of oxygen, so frequent rests are needed. Heavy weight training is considered anaerobic. The weight-training workout in this book utilizes light weights and becomes aerobic when you "speed-set," "giant-set," or "super-giant-set" (see page 55).

Forty-eight-Hour Recovery Principle: allowing forty-eight hours before rechallenging a muscle with a weight-training workout in order to allow the muscle optimum growth and to prevent overtraining and muscle attrition (wearing down).

Intensity of Workout: the degree of challenge of a given workout. You can increase the intensity of your workout by shortening or eliminating your rests and/or by raising your weights.

Metabolism: the chemical and physical process continually going on in the body, consisting of the process of changing food into fuel or energy, waste products, and living tissue. In simple terms, metabolism, or "basal metabolism," means the minimum quantity of energy you need to use to sustain life. After twelve weeks of doing this workout, you will increase your basal metabolism by about 15 percent and be able to eat about 15 percent more than you ate before without getting fat.

Muscle Isolation: the exercising of specific muscles and bones without using other muscles and bones. For example, when you do the palms-up wrist curl, you are isolating your wrist and forearm—and exercising the muscles and bones in those areas and not the muscles and bones in your biceps, shoulders, chest, thighs, and so on.

Non-split Routine: the exercising of the entire body on one workout day. If you opt to do the thirty-two-minute workout, you will do the non-split routine. However, if you do this, you must not work out with weights the next day because the muscles need forty-eight hours to recover. If you do any form of a split routine, you are not focusing on the same muscles the next day, so of course you can continue to work out with weights. Since the buttocks and abdominals do not require weights, they are an exception to the forty-eight-hour recovery principle.

Plateau: a weight ceiling, where one can choose to remain or attempt to break through. Most people reach their ideal weight-training plateau in about a year. If you are not happy with the size of your muscles and want them to be bigger, break through your plateau and keep going. I found that I needed to go up to ten-, fifteen-, and twenty-pound dumbbells. I'm happy here. I'll stay here forever.

Progression: adding weights to a specific exercise when the weight previously lifted becomes too easy. For example, you will be using one-, two-, and three-pound dumbbells to start with. But in a few weeks you may see that the one pounders are too easy and instead use two-, three-, and five-pound dumbbells. A few weeks later you may see that you can use three, five, and eight pounds, and yet a few weeks later you may be ready for five, eight, and ten—all the way up to eventually, say, ten-, fifteen-, and twenty-pound dumbbells. (That's where I'm at and where I'll stay! Why? See the previous term, "Plateau.")

Routine: the specific combination of exercises prescribed for a certain body part. For example, in this workout the back routine requires you to do the leaning one-arm dumbbell row, the back overhead pullover, and the double-arm upright row.

Split Routine: exercising a given number of body parts on one workout day and a given number of other body parts on another workout day. Split routines can vary by dividing the body into four parts, the way you will if you are on the minimum eight-minute plan, or by dividing the body into two parts, the way you will if you are on the sixteen-minute plan. (There are other ways to "split up" the workouts, but they are irrelevant here.)

Weight-Bearing Aerobics: activities that utilize the weight of the body. For more details, see page 155.

Workout: all the exercises you perform in a given day. The term can also refer to your entire workout—for example, every exercise in this book is your total "workout."

Muscle, Bone, and Appearance Expressions

Here are some terms regarding the improvement of muscle and bone.

Bone Density: the mass and solidity of the bone. Experts disagree over the age when natural peak bone mass is reached, but it is between twenty-five and thirty-five years of age.

Cellulite: the dimpled, craterlike fat that is formed by enlarged fat cells, which are joined together and attached to connecting fibrous tissue just beneath the surface of the skin. Cellulite appears on the thighs, stomach, and hip/buttocks areas (as well as arms and other body parts) on women and some men. Cellulite can be diminished and eventually eliminated by working out with weights and consuming a low-fat diet. As muscles are formed under the skin, and as excess fat is removed through diet, the bumpy surface eventually becomes smooth.

Definition: the delineated lines that separate muscles from each other, divide muscles themselves, and make them appear more shapely and appealing, giving the body a more balanced, symmetrical look. Your body will become defined as a side benefit of this workout.

Muscle Density: the hardness or solidity of a muscle. A muscle becomes denser as it increases in strength when challenged. The muscle becomes "toned" as opposed to flabby.

Muscle Mass: the size of a given muscle. You will experience very moderate muscle mass growth along with shaping and defining as you do this workout.

Skeleton: the structural framework of the human body—composed of 206 bones, which are controlled by muscles and nerve impulses. This workout will improve your entire skeleton and your posture as well.

Symmetry: the balance and proportion of each muscle in the body in relation to all the other muscles. This workout will improve your body symmetry by building moderate muscle mass where needed and giving ideal definition to your overall musculature.

Equipment for This Workout

Ankle Weight: a wraparound band that contains slotted spaces where various-sized weight inserts can be placed. You will use ankle weights for only one optional exercise in this workout—the leg extension. (You may choose not to do that exercise, in which case you will need only dumbbells for this workout.)

Barbell: a long bar that has various weights at either end; it is held in both hands. You will have the option of substituting a barbell for some of the exercises in this book. See "Machines, Etc." section.

Bench: a structure built specifically for weight-training exercises. It is long, narrow, and padded, and parallel to the floor.

Dumbbell: a handheld weight consisting of a short bar that has a raised section on either end. It can be held in one hand or both hands. Dumbbells are the only equipment you will need for this workout unless you choose the optional leg-extension exercise, which requires ankle weights.

Free Weights: weights that can be moved around and carried, as opposed to machines that are fixed and/or are too heavy to be carried about. Dumbbells and barbells are examples of free weights. You will be using dumbbells for this workout.

Machines: exercise equipment designed to challenge one or more specific body parts. Machines are operated in various ways: by air pressure, cams, pulleys, and so forth. You will be given the option of substituting machines for many of the exercises.

Step: a raised platform usually used for step aerobics but that can be used in place of a bench; it is raised at least 8 inches off the floor. You can substitute a step for a bench for this workout, although a bench is more comfortable.

Weight: the *resistance,* or the heaviness, of the dumbbell used in a given exercise. You will be using one-, two-, and three-pound weights (dumbbells) in each hand to start with. Note: When I say "one-pound dumbbells," I always mean "each dumbbell." Never add up the weights.

The Muscles and Bones in the Body, in the Order of the Workout Chapters

For your convenience, the following paragraphs will describe the muscles and the bones in the body in the same order as your workout chapters so that when you are working out, you can easily find them in this section. Look at the anatomy photographs and bone illustrations as you read the various descriptions, then locate them on your own body.

Back Muscles and Bones

The back muscles consist of two important areas: the **trapezius** and the **latissimus dorsi.**

The trapezius muscle is flat and shaped like a triangle. It begins at the spine and runs from the back of the neck down to the middle of the back. The function of the trapezius muscle is to shrug the shoulders, pull the head back, and support the shoulder blade when the arm is raised.

The "latissimus dorsi," or "lats," begin along the spinal column, in the middle of the back and toward the shoulders, and travel up to the front of the upper arm. These muscles pull the shoulder back and downward, and extend the arm. They give the back a **V** appearance, and when developed can make the waist look smaller.

The most important bones in the back are the **lumbar vertebrae,** found in the lower vertebral column, and the **sacrum** and **coccyx.**

The **vertebral column** (which we commonly call the "spine" or the "backbone") consists of twenty-five bones called the vertebrae. Seven of these bones are found in the neck area (cervical vertebrae), and twelve are found in the chest area (thoracic vertebrae). The lowest five, found in the small of the back, are called the lumbar vertebrae. The sacrum is formed by the fusion of five sacral vertebrae, and the coccyx is formed by the fusion of four coccygeal vertebrae. (Both the sacrum and the coccyx are located at the very bottom of the spinal column.)

All the back, abdominal, leg, hip/buttocks, and shoulder exercises help to strengthen and thicken the entire vertebral column. The back, abdominal, and hip/buttocks exercises especially help to strengthen the lumbar vertebrae, the sacrum, and the coccyx.

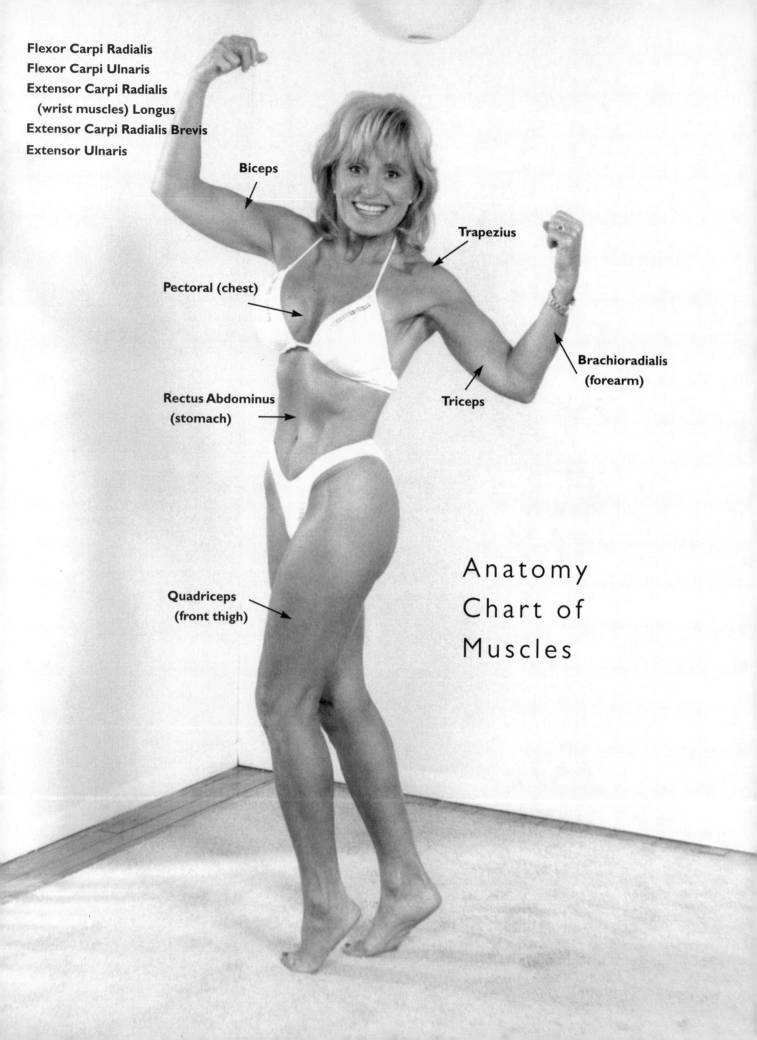

Flexor Carpi Radialis
Flexor Carpi Ulnaris
Extensor Carpi Radialis
   (wrist muscles) Longus
Extensor Carpi Radialis Brevis
Extensor Ulnaris

Biceps

Trapezius

Pectoral (chest)

Brachioradialis
(forearm)

Rectus Abdominus
(stomach)

Triceps

Quadriceps
(front thigh)

Anatomy
Chart of
Muscles

Deltoid
(shoulder)

Latissimus Dorsi (back)

Anatomy
Chart of
Muscles

Gluteus Maximus
Gluteus Medius
Gluteus Minimus (buttocks)

Sartoris/Adductor
(inner thigh)

Biceps Femoris
(back thigh)

Gastrocnemius (calf)

Abdominal (Rectus Abdominus) Muscles and Relevant Bones

The front abdominal area consists of a long, powerful, segmented muscle called the **rectus abdominus.** This muscle runs above and below the waist, and connects the pubic bones to the ribs and sternum, and along with other abdominal muscles, it helps to flex the vertebral column. The abdominal muscles pull the upper body toward the lower body when sitting up from a lying position.

When you strengthen the abdominal muscles, you provide support for your back muscles. For this reason I have grouped the back and abdominal workouts together.

The most important bones associated with the abdominal area are the bones discussed above, the vertebral column, specifically the lumbar vertebrae. All the abdominal exercises in this workout help strengthen the abdominal muscles and the backbone, and help support the back muscles. In addition, strong abdominal muscles help you to do all your exercises with more vigor, since the abdominal area is the "center of strength."

Leg Muscles and Bones: Thigh and Calf

The front thigh, or **quadriceps,** is composed of four muscles (hence *quadri*ceps). These muscles originate at the hip or thigh bones and meet at the knee. They serve to help you extend your leg from the bent position.

The inner thigh consists of the **sartoris** and **adductor** muscles. The sartoris muscle runs along the inner thigh, from the hipbone to the inside of the knee. This muscle is used to rotate the thigh. The adductor muscle originates from the lower pelvic area on the pubic bone and rises to the shaft of the thighbone, where it is inserted. This muscle helps to rotate, flex, and pull the legs together from a wide stance.

The back thigh is composed of the **biceps femoris,** a two-headed muscle, and the **semimembranosus** and **semitendinosus** muscles, or the "hamstrings." This muscle group works to bend the knee. These muscles originate in the bony area of the pelvis and terminate along the back of the knee joint.

The calf muscle, or **gastrocnemius,** is two-headed, and another muscle, the **soleus** muscle, lies just under it. These muscles connect in the middle of the lower leg and tie in with the Achilles tendon. The calf muscles work to help bend the knee and flex the foot downward.

The leg bones consist of the **femur** (thighbone), **patella** (knee bone), **tibia** (shinbone), and **fibula,** which connect to the ankle bones or **tarsals.**

The femur is the largest and strongest bone in the human body. It is attached to the pelvic girdle. It has a large rounded head, a neck, and two big protrusions to which the leg and buttocks muscles are attached. At the bottom end of the humerus, two rounded projections connect the bone to the shinbone (tibia). It is the upper section of the femur (the long thighbone) that breaks when doctors say one has a "hip fracture."

The kneecap, or patella, is connected to the lower femur. Of the bones running from the knee to the ankle, the tibia and fibula, the tibia is the thickest; the fibula, a thinner bone, is located beside the tibia.

The ankle is composed of seven tiny bones called **tarsals,** which join other bones, the **metatarsals** and **phalanges,** to form the foot.

All the leg exercises strengthen and build the muscle and bone of the entire leg area, including the thigh, knee, ankle, and foot, but thigh exercises specifically zone in on thigh muscle and bone, and calf muscle exercises zone in on calf muscle and bone.

Hip/Buttocks Muscles and Bones

The **gluteus maximus** is the largest muscle in the human body. It originates at the iliac crest of the thighbone and extends down the tailbone. This muscle works to extend and rotate the thigh when extreme force is needed, such as when you climb stairs. The **gluteus medius** lies just beneath the gluteus maximus and works to raise the leg out to the side and to balance the hips as you transfer your weight from one foot to the other. The **gluteus minimus** originates on the iliac crest of the hipbone and has the same function as the gluteus medius.

The hip/buttocks bones form the **pelvic girdle**—which is composed of two bones, called **pelvic bones.** These bones form a bowl-like structure that supports an area of the lower abdomen. Each of the two pelvic bones is composed of three bones—**ilium, ischium,** and **pubis**—which meet and form a cuplike socket called the **acetabulum,** at which point the top of the femur (thighbone) is attached.

All the hip/buttocks exercises work to tighten and strengthen the bones and muscles in the hip/buttocks area, but the leg exercises also help to do this.

Arm Muscles and Bones: Wrist and Forearms, Biceps, and Triceps

The muscles that help to flex the wrist run up through the forearm. The most significant muscles are the **flexor carpi radialis, flexor carpi ulnaris, extensor carpi radialis longus**, and **extensor carpi radialis brevis**. The wrist is extended and moved from side to side by the extensor carpi radialis longus and the extensor carpi radialis brevis, along with the **extensor carpi ulnaris.**

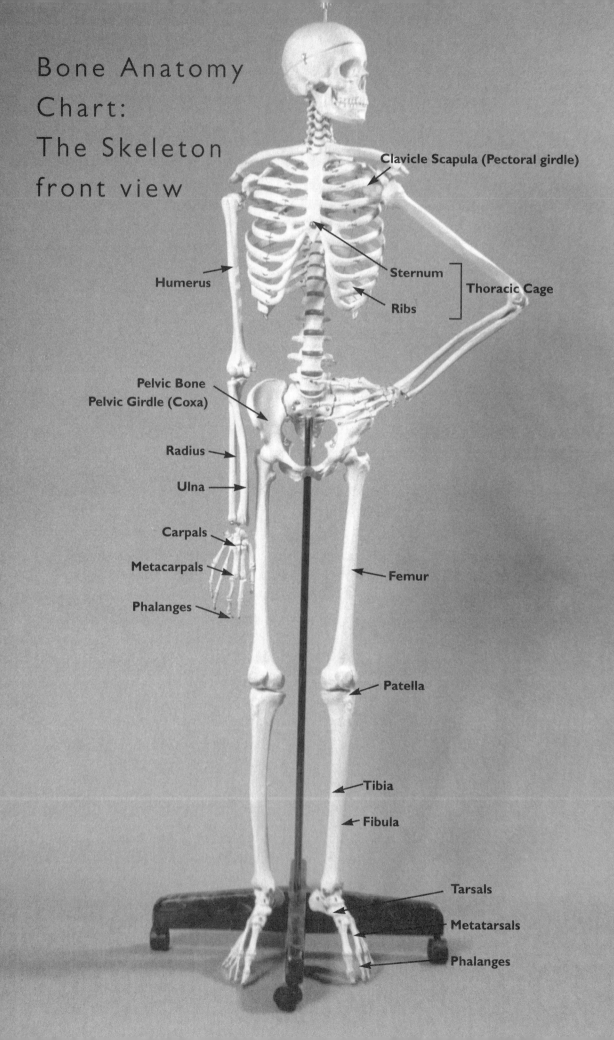

Bone Anatomy
Chart:
The Skeleton
front view

Clavicle Scapula (Pectoral girdle)

Humerus

Sternum

Ribs

Thoracic Cage

Pelvic Bone
Pelvic Girdle (Coxa)

Radius

Ulna

Carpals

Metacarpals

Phalanges

Femur

Patella

Tibia

Fibula

Tarsals

Metatarsals

Phalanges

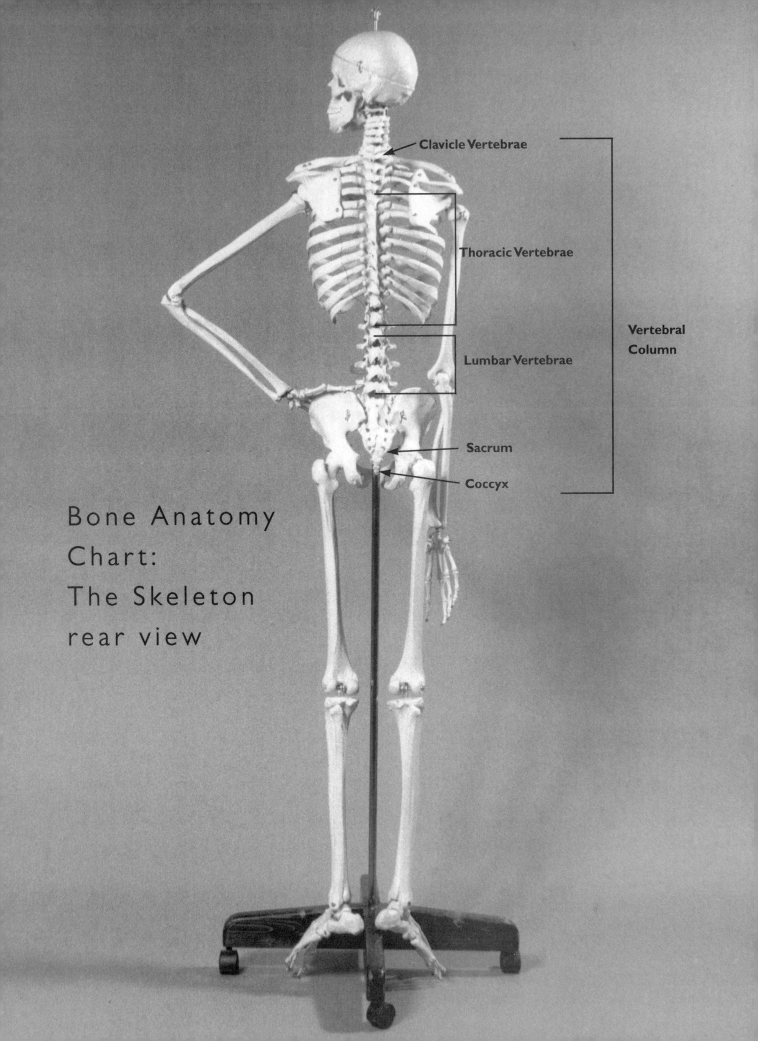

Clavicle Vertebrae

Thoracic Vertebrae

Lumbar Vertebrae

Vertebral Column

Sacrum

Coccyx

Bone Anatomy
Chart:
The Skeleton
rear view

The **brachioradialis,** a muscle that functions to flex the arm at the elbow, originates at the distal lateral end of the **humerus** bone and is attached to the lateral surface of the **radius.**

The bones of the wrist consist of the end points of the forearm bones, the radius and the **ulna,** joined by the small carpal bones lined up in two rows of four each.

The bones of the forearm consist of the ulna, which is located on the outer side of the arm (vertical to the pinky finger), and the radius, which is located on the inner side of the arm (vertical to the thumb). Both bones are attached to the upper arm bone, the humerus, and are connected at the elbow joint. The lower part of the ulna forms a major part of the wrist; hence the word "ulna" is sometimes used to indicate the wrist.

Both of the wrist exercises and all of the arm exercises, along with every exercise where you hold a weight in your hand, helps to strengthen and build the muscle and bone of the entire wrist and forearm area.

The **biceps muscle** originates at the shoulder blade and ends at the forearm. This muscle has two heads (which is why it's called *bic*eps). The hill of the biceps muscle is caused by the joining of these two heads. This muscle works to twist the hand and to flex the arm.

The **triceps muscle** originates at the shoulder blade and the upper arm, and inserts at the elbow. It has three heads (hence the term *tri*ceps). This muscle works to pull the arm back and to extend the arm and the forearm.

Both the biceps and triceps are undergirded by the long, strong humerus bone. At the higher end of the humerus bone you will find a smooth, rounded head and two small, round protrusions: the greater and lesser "tubercles," where muscles attach. All the biceps exercises specifically zone in on the biceps muscles, as do the triceps exercises for triceps, but the biceps and triceps exercises serve to strengthen and thicken the humerus bone as well as the wrist and forearm bones.

Shoulder (Deltoid) Muscles and Bones

The shoulder muscle is shaped like an upside-down Greek letter, "delta," hence the word "**deltoid.**" It consists of three parts: the front (anterior), side (medial), and rear (posterior) areas. This muscle originates in the upper area of the shoulder blade and collarbone, and is attached on the bone of the upper arm. The deltoid muscles function to lift the arm and move it forward, sideways, and backward.

The shoulder bones consist of the **scapula** and **clavicle** (called the **pectoral girdle**). (Note: It bothers me that the shoulder bones are called the "pectoral girdle" when we associate the word "pectoral" with chest. Perhaps they are so-named because they are located above the pectoral muscles.) The scapula has a socket at the end that holds the humerus (upper arm bone). The clavicle is shaped like a rod, and it braces the scapula against the top of the sternum, or breastbone. Muscles attach to both the scapula and the clavicle.

All the shoulder exercises work to strengthen and tighten the bone and muscle in the shoulder area. In addition, chest and arm exercises help strengthen these muscles.

Chest Muscles and Bones

The chest muscles are called the **pectoral muscles, pectoralis major,** or "pecs." These muscles look like a two-headed fan. The upper head (called the clavicular head) forms the upper pectoral area, and the larger head (called the sternal head) forms the lower pectoral area. These muscles originate at the collarbone and run along the sternum to the cartilage connecting the upper ribs to the sternum. This muscle helps to flex and abduct the arm.

The chest bones consist of the **thoracic cage,** which is composed of the **sternum (breastbone)** and **ribs.** All these bones serve as a protective cage for your heart, lungs, and other internal organs. The sternum consists of three parts: the **body,** a dagger-shaped structure attached to most of the ribs; the **manubrium,** the uppermost area; and the **xiphoid process,** the lowermost portion.

There are twelve pairs of ribs, but only the first seven are called "true ribs." Only these ribs are directly attached to the breastbone. The other five ribs are called "false ribs" because they are not directly attached to the breastbone.

All the chest exercises work to strengthen and shape the muscles and bones of the chest area. In addition, shoulder, abdominal, and arm exercises also help build and strengthen muscle and bone in this area.

Motivation to Work Out

Before we move to the next chapter, Creative Workouts, where you will learn how to use the material in this book for the ideal workout of your choice, let's get motivated.

Why bother to do the workout? Why not just relax and enjoy life and let nature take its course? Because nature did not intend for you to lie stagnant. Nature intended you to work—somewhat in the fashion of the caveman and cavewoman. But technology and modern science have tried to fool Mother Nature by making everything easy. In fact, you don't have to move out of your chair at all these days. You can just sit at your desk, surf the Internet, and run your word processor. The only body parts being exercised are your brain and your fingers. So in order to really let nature take its course, you must do some exercise; otherwise, you will be going against nature, and negative things will happen to you long before your time.

What would happen if you didn't exercise? Not only will you hate the way you look (but you already know that—flab, fat, the works), but your health will deteriorate. Your muscles and bones will atrophy, and you'll become weak and old before your time. Maintaining your diet is not enough! You could be "skinny fat" with porous, weak bones and flabby weak muscles. So you must incorporate exercise into your daily plan—specifically, weight-training exercise.

How to Find the Time

You must make an appointment with yourself to work out, and this appointment must be non-negotiable. You don't argue with yourself about brushing your teeth or taking a shower. You just do it. So it must be with exercise.

I'm asking you for a minimum of eight minutes a day. Don't tell me you can't afford that. The best thing to do is set up a work area in the corner of a room and do your workout the first thing in the morning—before you eat or dress for your day. Don't even think. After you've read this book, practiced the exercises (you can do this in the evenings or on the weekend), and set up your area, you just jump out of bed every morning and do your workout. After it becomes a habit, you may want to increase your workout to sixteen minutes.

You say you just can't do it every morning. Okay. Then do the thirty-two-minute workout only twice a week. One of your workouts can be on a weekend day. Since you must skip a day (see pages 53–54 for reasons), you'll have to do your second workout during the week. Either get up early or do it later in the day. (If you really want to go wild, you can even do the thirty-two-minute workout a third time during the week. This would be the absolute maximum. All of this is explained in chapter 4.)

When You're Tempted to Skip a Workout

What do you do when you get up and say, "I'm tired. I'm not in the mood. I'm late already. I work two jobs. The kids! My husband. My mother. I'm not doing it"? Discuss the following with yourself:

1. How will I feel later in the day after skipping a workout, as opposed to how I will feel later in the day after working out and keeping my promise to myself?

2. Who am I fooling? I have no choice. If I want to live a quality life by looking and feeling good, I must do this. I must not be immature and seek to please my immediate need to relax. I'll bite the bullet and do it. I'll respect myself for it.

3. What is an eight- to sixteen-minute time investment—considering all I'm getting back for it? Don't I waste more time on the telephone or watching TV? You can work out while watching TV if necessary. Cut your phone conversations down. Do it at lunchtime in your office with the door shut. Come what may, do it.

4. If I don't do it now, I'll have to squeeze it in later. Better to get it over with now.

Benefits of Making the Small Time Investment

You will not atrophy! You will stop trying to fool Mother Nature. You'll make up for the reality of the society we live in—technology laziness. In short, you'll live and thrive and look and feel younger, happier, and healthier than you've ever been in your life. I don't mean to brag, but look at me. I'm pushing fifty-five, and I look and feel better than I did in my twenties.

Just to remind you of all the benefits, I'm going to repeat my list from chapter 1, this time in a different order just in case these are your priorities. In fact, why don't you number the list in order of your priorities, one being the highest, and so on.

Loss of excess body fat, replaced with tight, toned muscles in twelve weeks

Increased metabolism so you burn more fat twenty-four hours a day

Reduced dress or pant size in three weeks

Toned, defined, firm, shapely body

Improved stamina: sports, life tasks, and you know what else (begins with _s_)

Increased strength—stronger muscles

Increased energy

Reduced stress level

Improved outlook on life, self-image, and self-confidence

Reduced pain from arthritis

Improved posture

Improved balance and agility

Increased bone density—stronger bones

Reduced pain from arthritis

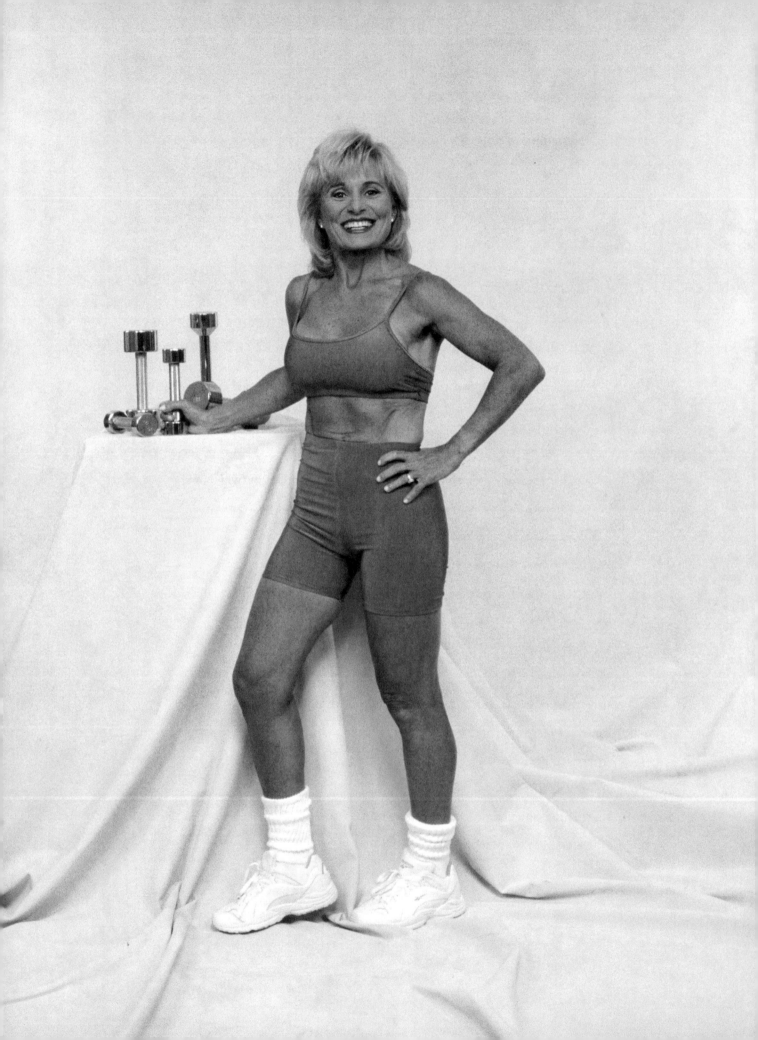

4. Creative Workouts

In this chapter you'll learn how to do the workout—and to ease into it—no matter what shape you are in. You'll also see whether you want to do the eight-, sixteen-, or thirty-two-minute plan, and learn how to use this book if you just want to strengthen and beautify certain body parts—and not bother with others. (But I warn you, I will try to motivate you to exercise your entire body.) You will find out how to exercise those body parts that are crucial to your athletic activity. I'll also show you how to do special extra work for troublesome body parts and how to intensify the workout so that you get even more out of it.

In addition, this chapter will explain which weights to use, when and how to increase them when they become too easy, how to use the machine alternatives, how to work in your aerobic exercises (detailed in chapter 9). It will also give specific suggestions for workout schedules and tell you how to maintain your strong, beautiful, fit body once you achieve it.

How to Do the Workout

You will use a very simple time-tested system for every exercise that utilizes weights—the pyramid system. As briefly explained on page 28, the pyramid system involves the adding of weight to each set, at the expense of a few repetitions. In the early stages of your workout, to ensure that you use proper form and don't injure yourself, you'll be using very unintimidating, light weights: one-, two-, and three-pound dumbbells (handheld weights). Note: This refers to each one whenever I refer to the weight of dumbbells. Here's how your beginning weight pyramid system will look.

> SET 1: 12 repetitions with 1-pound dumbbells; rest for 15–30 seconds
> SET 2: 10 repetitions with 2-pound dumbbells; rest for 15–30 seconds
> SET 3: 8 repetitions with 3-pound dumbbells; rest for 15–30 seconds

Technically speaking, the above is the "modified" pyramid system but is most effective for this workout.

How does it work? Let's use your first exercise, the leaning one-arm dumbbell row, as an example. You pick up your one-pound dumbbell and do *twelve* repetitions, looking at the photographs and following the exercise instructions. Since this is a one-arm-at-a-time exercise without resting, you will do twelve repetitions for the other side of your body.

You will rest fifteen to thirty seconds. Then you'll pick up your two-pound dumbbell and do *ten* repetitions for each side of your body. You'll again rest for fifteen to thirty seconds. Finally, you'll pick up your three-pound dumbbells and do *eight* repetitions for each side of your body.

What now? You don't stop there. You continue on to the next exercise, which is your back overhead pullover. You go through the same exact method, only this time you work both arms at one time. Boom-boom-boom—you do your three sets. Now you're moving along to the next exercise, the double-arm upright row—again, two arms at a time.

Okay. You've zipped through your back workout, but you're not finished yet. You have to keep going—right into your abdominal workout. But here you don't use any weights, and when you don't use any weights, you don't use the pyramid system!

Whenever you are not using weights, you do fifteen to twenty-five repetitions for each set. But you still do three sets. Here's how your sets and repetitions for hips/buttocks and abdominals will look.

> SET 1: 15–25 repetitions with no weight; rest for 15–30 seconds
> SET 2: 15–25 repetitions with no weight; rest for 15–30 seconds
> SET 3: 15–25 repetitions with no weight; rest for 15–30 seconds

Don't worry. You will be reminded in each exercise instruction how many sets and repetitions to do, what weights to use or not use, and how long and when to take your rests. Now let's continue your first day workout. You completed your back workout, and now you're ready to do your abdominal workout. You do fifteen to twenty-five repetitions of your first abdominal exercise, the crunch. You rest for fifteen to thirty seconds, and you do your second and third sets, again doing fifteen to twenty-five repetitions each. You then proceed to your next abdominal exercise, the bent-knee sewn lift. You do your three sets as above and proceed to your final abdominal exercise, the ceiling sewn lift, and do three sets. At this point you will have finished your workout for the day if you are on the eight-minute-a-day plan.

In any case, you will use the exact same method through your next three workout chapters—pyramiding whenever you use weight, and doing fifteen to twenty-five repetitions for each set for abdominals and hip/buttocks exercises.

What About Stretching?

Before you start the workout for each day, you will do a quick warm-up stretch to prepare you for the exercises. You can repeat the warm-up stretch two more times and/or lengthen it to twenty to thirty seconds if you wish, but that's optional except for certain warm-up stretches where I specifically ask you to repeat or lengthen the stretch.

Using the Warm-Up Exercise Stretches

You can use the warm-up exercise stretch to replace an exercise if you can't do certain ones. In this case, you will either pyramid the weights if a weight is required or do fifteen to twenty-five repetitions.

I'll use the leg extension warm-up stretch as an example. If you use it as a stretch, simply extend your legs out and hold for ten seconds. If you use it as an exercise, you'll use the ankle weights and add a little weight to each set, pyramiding the weights as you would for any other exercise that uses weights. If you use the lying crossover exercise stretch to replace an exercise, you will do three sets of fifteen to twenty-five repetitions.

But chances are you will not have to use the warm-up exercise stretches to replace an exercise because the exercises have been carefully formulated to ensure maximum ease and safety. If you are in doubt at all, check with your doctor.

You Will Be Led Along by the Eyes

Don't worry that you have to remember any of this! The stretches and exercises are in the exact order that you will do them. The instructions are crystal clear, and what's more, you are reminded in each exercise exactly how many sets and repetitions to do, which weights to use (if any), and how long to rest. It will be so simple after a time or two that you won't believe it.

The Tear-Out Wall Chart

Once you know what you're doing and no longer have to refer to the exercise instructions, you can use the handy tear-out wall chart—the overview reduced-sized photographs—so you can zip through your workout without having to flip pages. Some women tell me they like this even better than a video because they can work at their own pace using the chart. (The chart is located on pages 199–211.)

Overview of All the Exercises in the Workout

Before I break it down and tell you which exercises you will do on what day (which will depend on the plan you decide to do—eight, sixteen, or thirty-two minutes), let me give you an overview of all the exercises in your workout, because no matter which workout you choose, you will eventually do all the exercises. The difference will be how many you do in one day. (The eight-minute people will do one-fourth of them in a day and will have worked the entire body in four days. The sixteen-minute people will do half of them in a day and will have worked the entire body in two days. The thirty-two-minute people will do all of them in one day and will have worked their entire body in one day. More about this later.)

Here is how your workout will look:

Back and Abdominals Workout

WARM-UPS: back press knee raise, dinosaur curl
BACK EXERCISES
   1. Leaning one-arm dumbbell row
   2. Back overhead pullover
   3. Double-arm upright row
ABDOMINAL EXERCISES
   1. Crunch
   2. Bent-knee sewn lift
   3. Ceiling lift

Leg-Hip/Buttocks Workout

WARM-UPS: single-leg extension, lying crossover
LEG EXERCISES
   1. Leg curl
   2. Lunge
   3. Inner thigh sweep, or
   3a. wide leg semi-squat
   4. Standing calf raise
HIP/BUTTOCKS EXERCISES
   1. Alternate prone butt lift
   2. Lying butt lift
   3. Standing bent-knee back leg extension

Arms: Wrist, Biceps, and Triceps Workout

WARM-UPS: doggie paw wrist-forearm stretch, scratch-your-back biceps-triceps pull

WRIST EXERCISES

1. Palms-up wrist curl
2. Palms-down wrist raise

BICEPS EXERCISES

3. Standing simultaneous curl
4. Concentration curl

TRICEPS EXERCISES

5. Triceps kickback
6. Seated one-arm overhead triceps extension

Shoulder and Chest Workout

WARM-UPS: hug-your-head shoulder-back stretch, overhead towel chest stretch

SHOULDERS

1. Seated simultaneous dumbbell press
2. Easy-does-it side lateral
2a. Regular side lateral
3. Alternate front raise

CHEST

1. Dumbbell bench press
2. Easy-does-it push-up
2a. Regular push-up
3. Dumbbell fly

So there you have it—an overview of your entire workout, no matter the length of time you choose to work out. But now let's get to the specific daily work you will do, depending on how long you want to work out.

The Eight-Minute Workout

This is a very simple plan. You will do a "four-day split" routine. In other words, you will work something different every day for four days in a row. After four days, you will have exercised your entire body. Then you will repeat the four days. In eight days you will have exercised your entire body twice—just about the ideal minimum time required to get optimal results in muscle shaping and strengthening, and bone building.

How will you do this? It's spelled out for you. The workout chapters, 5 through 8, tell you what to do each day. Chapter 5 is your workout for day one: back and abdominals. Chapter 6 is your workout for day two: leg and hip/buttocks. Chapter 7 is your workout for day three: arms: wrist, biceps, and triceps. Chapter 8 is your workout for day four: shoulders and chest. Those chapters contain the instructions and photographs for the exercises you need to do, and in the exact order:

Workout Day One: Back and Abdominals Workout

WARM-UPS: back press knee raise, dinosaur curl

BACK EXERCISES

1. Leaning one-arm dumbbell row
2. Back overhead pullover
3. Double-arm upright row

ABDOMINAL EXERCISES

1. Crunch
2. Bent-knee sewn lift
3. Ceiling lift

Workout Day Two: Leg-Hip/Buttocks Workout

WARM-UPS: single-leg extension, lying crossover

LEG EXERCISES

1. Leg curl
2. Lunge
3. Inner thigh sweep or
3a. wide leg semi-squat
4. Standing calf raise

HIP/BUTTOCKS EXERCISES

1. Alternate prone butt lift
2. Lying butt lift
3. Standing bent-knee back leg extension

Workout Day Three: Arms: Wrist, Biceps, and Triceps Workout

WARM-UPS: doggie paw wrist-forearm stretch, scratch-your-back biceps-triceps pull

WRIST EXERCISES

    1. Palms-up wrist curl

    2. Palms-down wrist raise

BICEPS EXERCISES

    3. Standing simultaneous curl

    4. Concentration curl

TRICEPS EXERCISES

    5. Triceps kickback

    6. Seated one-arm overhead triceps extension

Workout Day Four: Shoulder and Chest Workout

WARM-UPS: hug-your-head shoulder-back stretch, overhead towel chest stretch

SHOULDERS

    1. Seated simultaneous dumbbell press

    2. Easy-does-it side lateral

    2a. Regular side lateral

    3. Alternate front raise

CHEST

    1. Dumbbell bench press

    2. Easy-does-it push-up

    2a. Regular push-up

    3. Dumbbell fly

You repeat the four days, and you take a day off from working out with weights. But what if you don't want to repeat but instead want to take a day off after you complete the four-day cycle? Fine with me! You won't lose a whole lot—just slow your workout down by one day. But, frankly, I'd rather you repeat the cycle twice before you rest a day. But what if you think (and chances are you will): "Hey, this is silly. I can do much more than eight minutes a day. I love this. Let me do more." Great. Here's the sixteen-minute workout.

The Sixteen-Minute Workout

This is just as simple a plan. You will do a "two-day split" routine. In other words, you will work one-half of your body on workout day one, and the other half of your body on workout day two. Then you will repeat the cycle. In only four days you will have exercised your entire body twice. You can either take a day off or repeat the cycle one more time so that in six days you will have exercised your entire body three times. This is the ultimate workout. I advise you to do it if you can.

But what if you decide to take a day off after exercising the body once or twice? That is perfectly fine. You will still make excellent progress, but the fewer days you take off, the better.

But what if you want to take a day off even sooner—after you've done only half of your body? That's okay, too. Just make sure you exercise your entire body at least twice a week. That's the rule of thumb.

How will you know how to split the body up into two days? It's quite simple. You do chapters 5 and 6 for workout day one (back and abdominals, leg and hip/buttocks). On workout day two, you will do chapters 7 and 8 (arms: wrist, biceps, and triceps, and shoulder and chest). Here is what your workout will look like:

Workout Day One: Back and Abdominals Workout

WARM-UPS: back press knee raise, dinosaur curl
BACK EXERCISES
1. Leaning one-arm dumbbell row
2. Back overhead pullover
3. Double-arm upright row

ABDOMINAL EXERCISES
1. Crunch
2. Bent-knee sewn lift
3. Ceiling lift

Leg-Hip/Buttocks Workout

WARM-UPS: single-leg extension, lying crossover
LEG EXERCISES
1. Leg curl
2. Lunge
3. Inner thigh sweep or
3a. wide leg semi-squat
4. Standing calf raise

HIP/BUTTOCKS EXERCISES
1. Alternate prone butt lift
2. Lying butt lift
3. Standing bent-knee back leg extension

Workout Day Two: Arms: Wrist, Biceps, and Triceps Workout

WARM-UPS: doggie paw wrist-forearm stretch, scratch-your-back biceps-triceps pull

WRIST EXERCISES

1. Palms-up wrist curl
2. Palms-down wrist raise

BICEPS EXERCISES

3. Standing simultaneous curl
4. Concentration curl

TRICEPS EXERCISES

5. Triceps kickback
6. Seated one-arm overhead triceps extension

Shoulder and Chest Workout

WARM-UPS: hug-your-head shoulder-back stretch, overhead towel chest stretch

SHOULDERS

1. Seated simultaneous dumbbell press
2. Easy-does-it side lateral
2a. Regular side lateral
3. Alternate front raise

CHEST

1. Dumbbell bench press
2. Easy-does-it push-up
2a. Regular push-up
3. Dumbbell fly

You repeat the cycle (ideally one or two more times), then take a day off from weight training. Okay, I can read your mind: What if you want to do your entire body in one day? That's where we get to the thirty-two-minute workout.

The Thirty-Two-Minute Workout

The good news is that if you're "up for it"—that is to say, if you feel you have the energy and the motivation to do it—you can work your entire body in one day. You simply do everything—all the workout chapters 5, 6, 7, and 8, and all the body parts: back and abdominals; legs and hip/buttocks; arms: wrist, biceps, and triceps; and shoulders and chest—in one day. But there is a catch—actually, a good one. You must—and I repeat, *must*—take a day off from working out with weights the next day. Why? In chapter 3 I discussed the forty-eight-hour recovery period: When you are using weights, you must let the muscles rest for forty-eight hours before you stimulate them again. They need that time to recuperate; otherwise, you may overtrain them and wear them down rather than build them.

But how come we can work out eight days in a row with the eight-minute workout and six days in a row with the sixteen-minute workout? The answer is simple: You are not doing the same body parts two days in a row! As you may recall, each workout day exercises different body parts. Since here you will be doing your entire body in one day, if you worked out with weights the next day, you would be violating the forty-eight-hour recovery rule.

But you can do something on that "rest" day. You can work out without weights. You can do your aerobic exercises. Later in this chapter I'll explain how to incorporate them into your workout. You can also do extra stomach or hip/butt work, since these body parts do not use weights.

How will your thirty-two-minute workout look? Exactly the same as you read above when I gave you the overview of the whole workout. You'll simply do the whole workout, so I won't repeat it here.

Save Time and Burn More Fat by "Giant-Setting"

After you become very familiar with the workout and are doing it with ease, you may want to "giant-set," as described on page 28. Simply put, to giant-set you would do your first set of each exercise for a given body part without taking a rest. After resting for fifteen seconds, you do your second set for each exercise for that body part without taking a rest. You would then rest fifteen seconds and complete your final set for that body part. Let's take a look at how it works for the back. (It would be the same method for all body parts.)

WARM-UPS: back press knee raise, dinosaur curl
BACK EXERCISES
1. Leaning one-arm dumbbell row
2. Back overhead pullover
3. Double-arm upright row

Do your warm-up as usual. Then proceed to do your first set of twelve repetitions of the leaning one-arm dumbbell row with the one-pound dumbbells and, without resting, do your first set of the back overhead pullover with the one-pound dumbbells. And again without resting, do your first set of the double-arm upright row with the one-pound dumbbells. Now take a fifteen-second rest.

Do your second set of the leaning one-arm dumbbell row of ten repetitions using the two-pound dumbbells. Without resting, proceed to your back overhead pullover and do ten repetitions with the two-pound dumbbells. Once again without resting, proceed to your double-arm dumbbell row and perform ten repetitions with the two-pound dumbbells. Now rest for fifteen seconds.

Finally, do your third and last set of each exercise. You do eight repetitions of the leaning one-arm dumbbell row using the three-pound dumbbells and, without resting, you do eight repetitions of the back overhead pullover using the three-pound dumbbells. Again without resting, and using the three-pound dumbbells, do eight repetitions of the double-arm bent row.

What is the advantage of giant-setting? The workout just zips by. It's over before you know it. You cut your rest time by two-thirds and in the process burn more fat!

(Note: When you come across a body part, such as the wrist, biceps, and triceps, that has only two exercises, simply do them two at a time instead of three at a time. This method would be called "super-setting" instead of "giant-setting.")

Equipment Needed for This Workout

All you will need for this workout, to start, are three sets of dumbbells (handheld weights), a chair with a back, a towel, a mat (if you don't have carpeted floors), and a bench (or a "step" like that used in step aerobics).

Start out by purchasing three sets of dumbbells: ones, twos, and threes. As mentioned before, I'm talking about the pounds for each weight, not together. This means you will hold a one-pound dumbbell in each hand, then a two-pound dumbbell in each hand, then a three-pound dumbbell. Where will you buy these weights? Look in the yellow pages under "Exercise Equipment" and call around. Ask: "Do you sell dumbbells? How much are they by the pound?" You should be able to purchase inexpensive iron dumbbells for about fifty cents a pound. This means that to get started you will need to spend only about $6.00—since your total weights will weigh only twelve pounds.

But watch out! Don't waste your money on fancy colored ones—unless, of course, you don't mind the expense and want to look at pretty weights. Also beware of the "sets" that you have to take apart; yours should be all ready for use. There won't be time to finagle with adjusting weights. Why do that when you can have separate sets for fifty cents a pound? But don't buy only three sets to begin with. Buy a few extra sets, because you're going to get strong faster than you can imagine. Buy a set of fives, eights, and tens, too! This leads me to my next important point.

Raising Your Weights When They Get Too Easy

You will start out by using very light weights, but after a week or two you may be ready for heavier ones. It will depend on how strong you were to begin with and how your particular muscles and bones respond to the workout. In any case, don't rush it. But when the weights feel too easy—when you know you can get many more reps than you're being asked to do—it's time to raise the weights.

Here's how to use the pyramid system while raising the weights.

BEGINNING WEIGHTS

SET 1: one-pound dumbbells
SET 2: two-pound dumbbells
SET 3: three-pound dumbbells

RAISING WEIGHTS THE FIRST TIME

SET 1: two-pound dumbbells
SET 2: three-pound dumbbells
SET 3: five-pound dumbbells

RAISING WEIGHTS THE SECOND TIME

SET 1: three-pound dumbbells
SET 2: five-pound dumbbells
SET 3: eight-pound dumbbells

RAISING WEIGHTS THE THIRD TIME

SET 1: five-pound dumbbells
SET 2: eight-pound dumbbells
SET 3: ten-pound dumbbells

RAISING WEIGHTS THE FOURTH TIME

SET 1: eight-pound dumbbells
SET 2: ten-pound dumbbells
SET 3: twelve-pound dumbbells

RAISING WEIGHTS THE FIFTH TIME

SET 1: ten-pound dumbbells
SET 2: twelve-pound dumbbells
SET 3: fifteen-pound dumbbells

RAISING WEIGHTS THE SIXTH TIME

SET 1: ten-pound dumbbells
SET 2: fifteen-pound dumbbells
SET 3: twenty-pound dumbbells

RAISING WEIGHTS THE SEVENTH TIME

SET 1: twelve-pound dumbbells
SET 2: fifteen-pound dumbbells
SET 3: twenty-pound dumbbells

How high will you eventually go? I stopped at ten, fifteen, and twenty pounds. You can decide where you want to stop. Just look at your body in the mirror and see if you're happy with the muscle development you've achieved. Most women I know don't go beyond twenty pounds for their highest dumbbell weight.

Different Weights for Different Exercises—After a While!

In the beginning, even if you find certain body parts stronger than others, I want you to use only the very light one-, two-, and three-pound dumbbells. After a few weeks, however, you will find that you simply can't stand doing stronger, larger muscles, such as the chest, with such light weights. You may be able to use higher weights for the chest. On the other hand, you may find that your shoulders are still too weak to raise the weights. By all means, raise only your chest—and, with it, maybe your biceps, back, and legs, which are other strong body parts. Triceps may linger behind with your shoulders. In time, you will absolutely raise the weights for even the weaker body parts—and perhaps all the way up to twelve, fifteen, and twenty. But take it easy. Don't rush. Let it happen naturally—but don't hold yourself back, either.

What About the Machine Alternatives and the Weights Used?

You will note that every exercise instruction notes a machine alternative in case you have a home-gym machine or want to work out in a fitness center utilizing the machines.

When it comes to deciding which pound weights to use, you will have to try each machine individually. The general rule is to start with little or no weight for your first set, raise it very slightly for your second set, and just a bit more for your final set. Then as you get stronger, increase the weights.

Machines and dumbbells use completely different systems of calculation. For example, when you have ten pounds on the lat pulldown machine, which exercises your back, it will feel as if you're using a three-pound dumbbell. Twenty pounds will feel like five pounds. Fifty pounds will feel like ten or fifteen pounds. Air pressure machines are a world unto themselves. You simply press the air button to increase the "weight." You "feel" it out, and you watch the needle on the weight-gauge go up higher.

No need to get into detail here. Just follow the general rule, but don't get hung up on numbers. Each machine is different and uses its own calculation system. As long as you are pyramiding your weights (adding to each set) and remembering to go heavier as you get stronger and the weights are too easy, you'll get the maximum benefit from the workout.

Dumbbells Versus Machines

In general, dumbbells are better than machines for a variety of reasons. First, they are quite versatile. You can do hundreds of different exercises with one simple set of dumbbells but only a few exercises on any given machine. You would need many expensive machines to equal what you can do with an inexpensive set of dumbbells. In addition, dumbbells force you to do all the work. With a machine you can drop the weight or raise it much more easily than with dumbbells. In addition, machines are made for the "average-sized" person. Even though there are adjustments, it's very difficult to position the machine exactly for your body. Dumbbells, on the other hand, can be positioned to fit your exact needs. Another advantage of dumbbells is their convenience. You can keep them anywhere; they don't take up much space.

Machines do have some advantages over dumbbells. If you're working at a machine and drop the weight, the machine will catch it. You won't hurt yourself. In addition, some machines allow you to exercise certain body parts that need heavier weight and would be difficult to do with dumbbells. One is the lat pulldown machine, where you can do lat pulldowns for your back and, in addition, triceps pushdowns and overhead extensions for your triceps. (See machine alternatives if you want to do these.) The leg extension and leg curl machines are also useful; you can safely exercise your front and back thighs with heavier weights than you could with ankle weights or dumbbells because of the way these machines allow you to brace your back as you work.

The leg press machine, which positions you safely, allows you to use the kind of weight necessary for developing a significant front thigh muscle. You lie on your back as you work, so your back is protected. You could never use such heavy weights safely doing squats with free weights or even using a squat machine. The leg press machine is often used by people with problem backs or knees who want front thigh shaping and toning but cannot do squats or lunges.

Another machine I like is the seated calf machine because you can use heavy weights safely and develop significant calf muscles. You can go just so far by using your own body weight, by standing, or by holding a dumbbell on your lap while doing a seated calf raise. The machine allows you to sit in a safe position and raise fifty or more pounds without straining yourself.

Other machines not mentioned here are fine for working out. (See the "Machines, Etc." section of each exercise instruction if you're a "machine person" or want to use them for variety.)

If you decide to use the machine alternatives, all you have to do is go to the appropriate machine, read the machine instruction card, and/or ask the gym instructor to get you started. I do have three books that show you how to use machines: *Weight Training Made Easy*, *Now or Never*, and *Top Shape*. (See bibliography for more details.)

Now let's talk about workout schedules.

Workout Schedules for the Eight-Minute Workout

Note the strange "eight-day week" for the purposes of our workout. Also note the abbreviations:

bk/ab for back and abs

lg-hp/bt for legs and hip/buttocks

ch/sh for chest and shoulders and off wt to indicate days you will not be working out with weights.

MON.	TUES.	WED.	THURS.	FRI.	SAT.	SUN.	MON.
bk/ab	lg-hp/bt	arms	ch/sh	bk/ab	lg-hp/bt	arms	ch/sh

You take a day off on Tuesday and begin again.

Another way to do the workout is to do the full cycle Monday through Thursday, take a day off, then repeat the cycle. Just keep doing the four-day cycle, taking a day off and repeating the cycle. Can you instead keep repeating the eight-day cycle without taking a day off? Yes, but you may rebel out of boredom. Use your own judgment.

Workout Schedules for the Sixteen-Minute Plan

MON.	TUES.	WED.	THURS.	FRI.	SAT.	SUN.
bk/ab	arms	bk/ab	arms	bk/ab	arms	off wt
lg-hp/bt	ch/sh	lg-hp/bt	ch/sh	lg-hp/bt	ch/sh	

This is the maximum plan, where you work your entire body three times a week. The regular plan allows you to work your body two times a week. It would look something like this:

MON.	TUES.	WED.	THURS.	FRI.	SAT.	SUN.
bk/ab	arms	off wt	bk/ab	arms	off wt	off wt
lg-hp/bt	ch/sh		lg-hp/bt	ch/sh		

You could actually work any four days of the week to complete your regular sixteen-minute-a-day plan—even four days in a row—but why do that unless your schedule demands it? It's always better to spread it out if you can.

The Thirty-Two-Minute Plan

MON.	TUES.	WED.	THURS.	FRI.	SAT.	SUN.
Entire Workout		Entire Workout		Entire Workout		

It's that simple. The only catch here is that, no matter what, you should not do your entire workout two days in a row! Remember, the forty-eight-hour recovery period is very important when working out with weights. You must take a day off from weights in between workouts when you work your entire body.

But you can do something on the off days and even on the "on" weight-training days: aerobics.

Working Aerobics into Your Weight-Training Schedule

It's a good idea to do aerobics in addition to this workout. Aerobics are great for increasing heart and lung capacity, and therefore can help you do this workout more easily and help burn additional fat. The kind of "weight-bearing" aerobics you will be doing will also enhance bone density.

You can do your aerobic activities on your days off from weight-training, and on some days on, as long as you get a minimum of three days a week! Why a minimum of three days? Experts feel you should do aerobics at least three days a week in order to get the full heart-lung benefit.

If you really want to burn extra fat, you can do aerobics six days a week or even do them nonstop for a month. But if you're going to do aerobics nonstop, you'd better not do the same thing every day. It may take a toll on your joints and muscles. For example, if you run one day and walk the next, you may get away with doing aerobics for a month or more before your body demands a day off. Or even better, if you add a third element into the mix—stair stepping, say—or even a fourth, aerobic dance, you may be able to do aerobics on and on without taking a day off.

So how do you work aerobics into the above schedule? Here are some general rules regarding aerobics:

1. If you're not weight training on certain days, do aerobics on those days so that your body will not lie stagnant.

2. If you are doing aerobics on the same day as weight training, do them first if possible, so they can serve as a warm-up. If you have only a limited time, however, and it's a choice between weight training and aerobics, always do your weight training first. You can squeeze in your aerobics anytime later, but if you skip them, you won't lose as much as you would if you had skipped weight training.

3. Do aerobics a minimum of three days a week.

4. Do aerobics anytime, any day, whether you're weight training or not. There is no hard-and-fast "recovery rule" when it comes to aerobics.

5. Take off one day a week from aerobics. If you alternate aerobic activities, play it by ear. You may not want to take a day off. See chapter 9 for a discussion of various appropriate aerobic choices.

Note: Don't carry dumbbells or use ankle or wrist weights while doing aerobic activities. You can't reshape any body part that way, and you can injure yourself!

Special Workouts

Suppose you are engaged in a particular sport and want to know which exercises will enhance your strength and agility. Or suppose you are worried about osteoporosis and want to work only the body parts that are most vulnerable to fracture. I'll tell you which exercises help the most for your particular purpose, but it is better for you to do the total-body workout than simply pick and choose exercises for your sport. The body needs total muscle strength balance in order to have the greatest insurance against injury. In addition, you look so much better with total symmetry.

The workout chapters in this book are in order of importance for prevention of injury due to osteoporosis. The three most vulnerable fracture points when bones begin to thin are the lower back, the hip (actually the upper leg), and the wrist. You will see that chapter 5 deals with the first most vulnerable area, the back (and the supporting abdominals). Chapter 6 deals with the next most vulnerable spot, the legs and hip/buttocks area. Chapter 7 covers the third most vulnerable spot, the arms—which includes the wrist.

Does this mean you should leave out chapter 8, shoulders and chest? Absolutely not. But if you are concerned only with the most vulnerable fracture spots, you should know that these chapters focus on them.

Now let's talk about individual sports and activities, and which "workouts" are most important for them.

Tennis, Racquetball, Handball, Volleyball, Squash
Arms, legs, hip/buttocks, back, abdominals, and shoulders

Golf
Shoulders, back, abdominals, arms, and hip/buttocks

Running, Walking
Legs, hip/buttocks, abdominals, and back

Bike Riding

Legs, hip/buttocks, and back

Cross-Country Skiing, Downhill Skiing, Waterskiing

Legs, hip/buttocks, back, abdominals, shoulders, and arms

Swimming

Back, chest, shoulders, arms, hips, legs

Horseback Riding

Legs, hip/buttocks, back, shoulders

Martial Arts, Aerobic Dance, Ballroom Dancing, Social Dancing

Every single body part in this workout!

Now let's get to the special work for those who want to improve the look of certain body parts. You can devote extra workout time without unbalancing the body because certain body parts actually require more work in order to get into ideal shape.

You guessed the parts: the stomach and hip/buttocks areas!

Extra Work for Troublesome Body Parts

You can do your abdominal and hip/buttocks workout any day of the week—up to six days a week—adding them in on weight-training days when you are working other body parts. You may wonder if this is a contradiction of the forty-eight-hour recovery principle? It isn't. Remember I said that you must rest those body parts that work with weights? With the abdominal and hip/buttocks exercises, no weights are used, so you can give them extra exercises without negative consequences.

By spending more workout days on these body parts, you will tighten, tone, and define them more quickly and more intensely. But you may not want to do them as often as six days a week. Try to do them at least three or four days a week if you want to speed up your progress. But don't worry. Even if you do them the minimum, you'll still see marked improvement.

Personal Trainers

Think of me as your personal trainer. My goal is for you to be totally self-sufficient. I don't want you to have to pay good money time after time or to depend on someone else's energy to work out. If you feel you must do it, however, there's no harm in hiring a qualified personal trainer to take you through this workout once or twice, although it really isn't necessary. But beware. Personal trainers make their living on your needing them on a regular basis. So don't be surprised if your trainer tries to keep you working with him or her. That's all well and good if you enjoy it and can afford it, and if you feel your personal trainer is not holding you back.

Maintaining Your Strong, Beautiful Body

Okay. You've been doing the workout for six months. Your body looks and feels great. You're "in shape." Now what? Do you have to do this for the rest of your life? Yes! And why not? Your body is as dependent on exercise for health as it is for food! The only difference is, if you deprive your body of food, you die sooner than if you deprive your body of exercise. So stop thinking "When can I stop?" and start thinking of exercise as a new lifetime habit. If you get bored with this workout, try one of the workout books or videos listed on page 193 the bibliography.

If after a few months you still don't like working out, just think of it the way you do brushing your teeth or taking a shower—a "must be done, get it out of the way" activity. After a while you'll do it automatically.

You can always manage to find eight to sixteen minutes a day for working out. There's really no excuse for avoiding it. You can get up ten minutes earlier no matter how early you're getting up now, or you can work out while you're watching the news (if you must; I'd rather you concentrated on your workout). You can give up some talking on the telephone or reading of newspapers. Do whatever you must to get your workout in. It's worth the investment in health and beauty.

Taking Time Off from Working Out

Am I saying that you can never take a week or two off from working out? No. In fact, you can take a week off every six months without consequences. And when you do take off, don't stagnate. Be active. Move around. Enjoy your fit body by trying out new activities. If you're on vacation, for example, go skin-diving, parasailing, and so on.

What if you have to take off a few months or more because of an injury? Well, ask your doctor what you can do, and do it. He may say you can work certain body parts but not others. The idea is to "work around it." Do the best you can. Think of yourself as an athlete in training when you have an injury. Make it work *for* you rather than *against* you.

Changing the Order of the Exercises

What if you want to change the order of the exercises? Well, you can do it, but there are certain rules. You can change the order of the exercises within a given body part but not among body parts. In chapter 5, for example, back and abdominals, you can do any back exercise in any order, but don't start mixing in back with abs and then jumping to chapter 6 and mixing in legs and hip/buttocks at random. The rule is to either follow my exact order of the exercises or change the order only within a given body part.

What about changing the body parts within a given workout day? You can do that if you want. On workout day one, you are exercising back and abdominals, with the back first. There is no reason that you can't do abdominals first. The same holds true no matter what body parts you are exercising.

Getting More Out of the Workout by Increasing the Intensity

There are three ways to get more out of the workout.

1. After you know what you're doing, shorten or eliminate the rests. You burn more fat this way and get an aerobic workout in the bargain. If you do this, though, you will have to increase your weights more slowly.

2. Use heavier weights. (You build more muscle and bone this way.)

3. Flex throughout the movement. You get harder muscles this way. (You will note that I continually remind you when to flex and when to feel the stretch while you're working out.)

Easy-Does-It Break-in Plan

Unless you are a seasoned weight trainer, you should ease into your weight-training workout rather than try to go at it full force. Otherwise, you'll probably be so sore the next day, you'll want to quit. So do yourself a favor and invest the few weeks it will take to break in gently.

> WEEK 1: Do only the first set of each exercise.
> WEEK 2: Do the first and second sets of each exercise.
> WEEK 3: You are on the full program!

Since you are using such light weights, you can be in the full program after only two weeks! Isn't that wonderful? Diet and diet maintenance will be discussed in chapter 10.

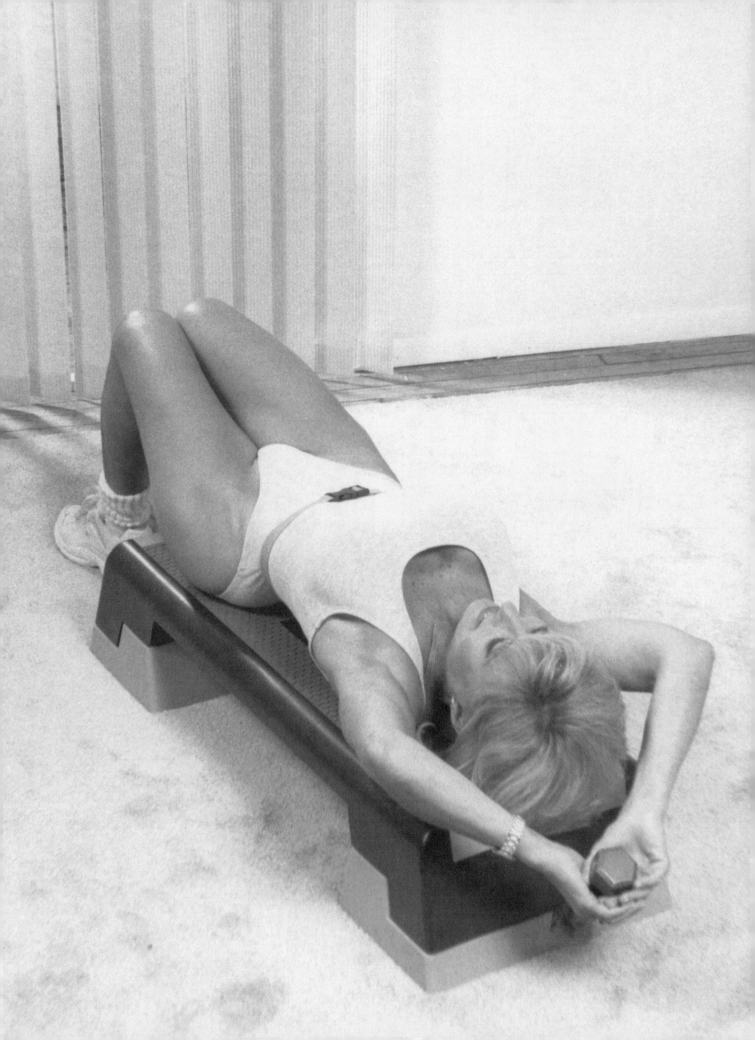

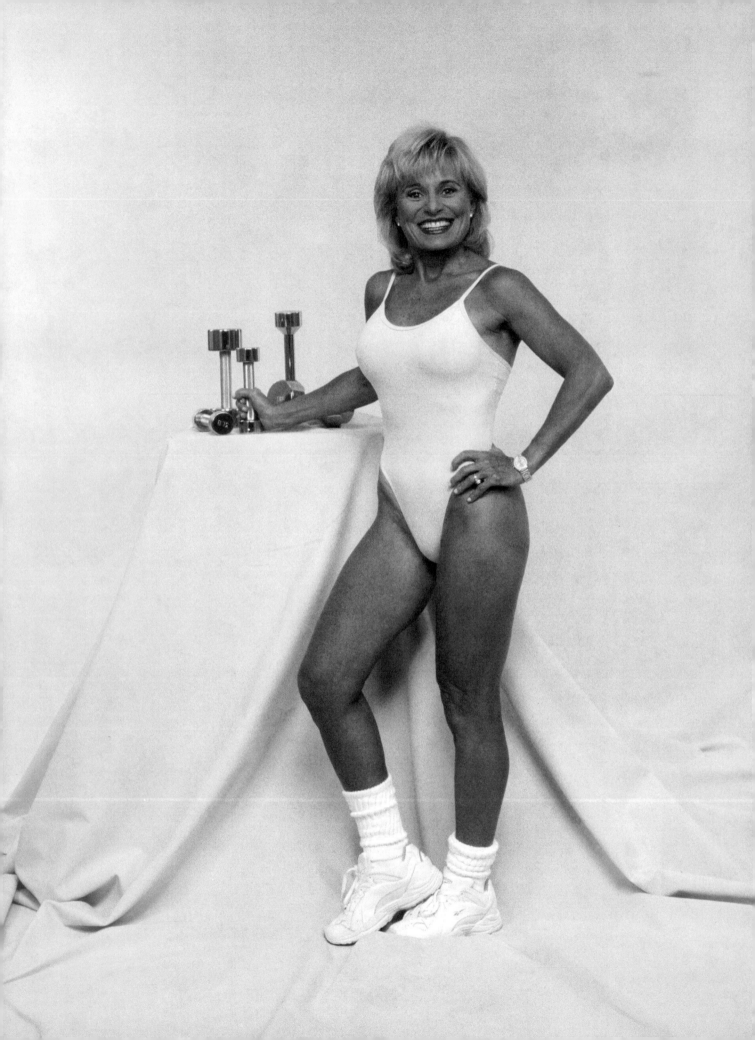

5. Back and Abdominals for Muscle Tone, Beauty, Bone, and Strength

Why do we group the back and abdominal areas together? The medical community agrees that they are closely linked when it comes to strength and posture. Weak abdominal muscles will further aggravate back problems, while strong abdominal muscles will help a weaker back. The first thing your doctor will tell you if you have a "bad back" is to start strengthening your abdominal muscles.

This chapter discusses exercising first your back, then your abdominal muscles and underlying bones. For a detailed description and anatomy photographs, see pages 38 and 39. It's a good idea to refer to the photographs and then locate the muscles and bones in your own body. As you work out, you can continually "tell" your muscles and bones to strengthen, reshape, and evolve into their optimum form.

The back muscles we'll be emphasizing here are the **trapezius** (located in the area of the shoulder, back, neck, and down the back) and the **latissimus dorsi** (located along the spinal column in the middle of the back and toward the shoulders), that travel up to the front of the upper arm. The bones that you'll be focusing on are the **lumbar vertebrae** (in the lower vertebral column), the **sacrum,** and **coccyx** (located on the lower end of the vertebral column). It is especially important to strengthen these bones because their location—your lower back—makes them extremely vulnerable to fracture. In fact, the spine is one of the top three fracture spots when bones begin to thin. It is composed of flat bones that are made of a higher percentage of soft "trabecular," or spongy, material, as opposed to the harder cortical material discussed on page 17.

You will exercise your entire abdominal muscle, or **rectus abdominus** (which runs above and below the waist and connects to the pubic bones, ribs, and chest). Your abdominal exercises will also work to strengthen the bones in the **vertebral column,** including the lumbar vertebrae. Note: The abdominal muscles located above the waist are called "upper abdominals," and those below the waist are called "lower abdominals," although technically speaking the abdominal muscle is really one long, segmented muscle.

Before I tell you the next fact, I want you to put on your "sunny" glasses and read with optimism. Now to the cold hard facts: More than one-third of women over sixty-five experience a fracture of one of the vertebrae in the back. If bones are thinning, it can happen so easily, by making a sudden move or mildly tapping the bone in a light bang or fall. Such fractures are called "crush" fractures because the vertebra is compressed. In this event, you will have severe pain that lasts for weeks. But this isn't going to happen to you because you are wisely taking steps to strengthen your bones (even if you're doing this workout for beauty).

Now for the interesting part. One of the first things doctors recommend when a crush fracture occurs, after a healing period, is exercise to strengthen the back and abdominal muscles. So let's get busy *before* the problem occurs, but be comforted that there is something we can do to help ourselves no matter what has already happened.

You will do one set of the warm-up stretch (unless you are substituting it for an exercise) and three sets of each exercise, using the pyramid system. You will be reminded in each exercise instruction about sets, reps, weights, and rests, but for a fuller explanation, you can review chapter 4.

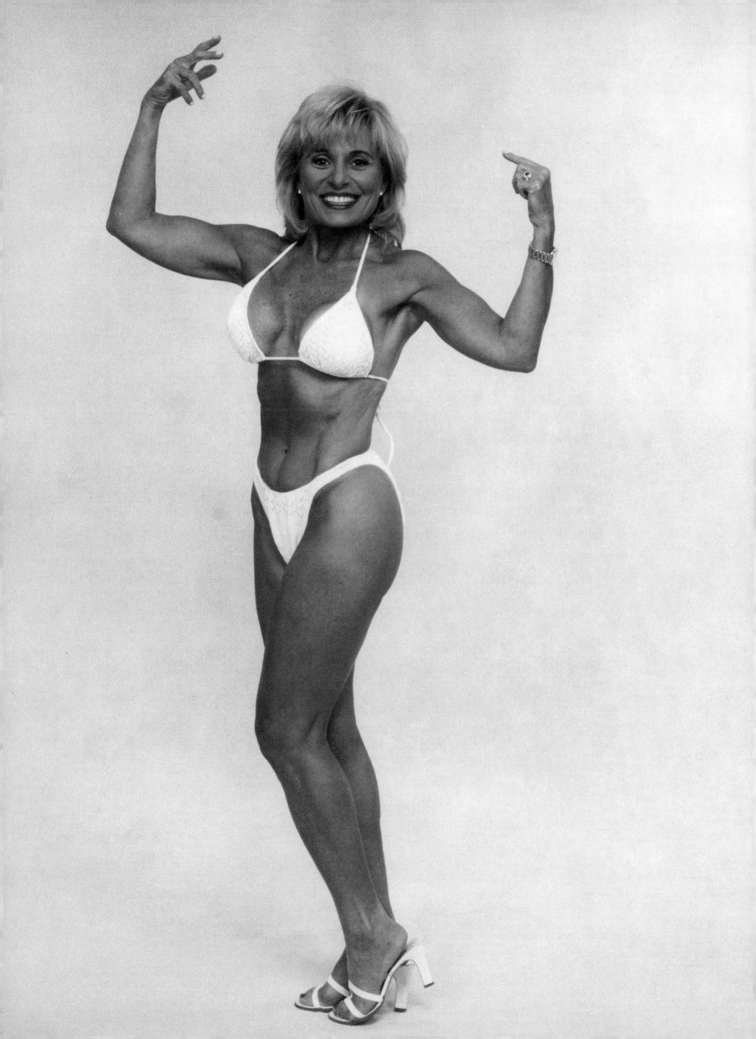

Warm-Up #1: Back Press Knee Raise

This two-part exercise stretch relaxes and strengthens the entire spinal column—especially the lower (lumbar), sacral, and coccyx areas.

POSITION

Lie flat on your back on a mat or rug with your knees bent, holding your knees as close to your chest as possible. (Feel the stretch in your spinal column. You have already done the first part of the stretch!)

ACTION

Place the soles of your feet flat on the ground, place your hands behind your neck, and press your back flat into the mat by tightening your buttocks and abdominal muscles. Hold for five seconds and release. Return to the start position and repeat two more times. Feel the tension release from your lower back.

TIPS

Don't hold your breath. Breathe naturally. Relax and enjoy the stretch. You may be tempted to repeat this stretch a few more times. If you do, don't fight the feeling! It's worth the investment of a few more seconds.

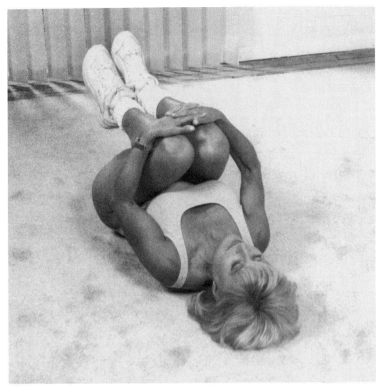

BACK PRESS KNEE RAISE: START

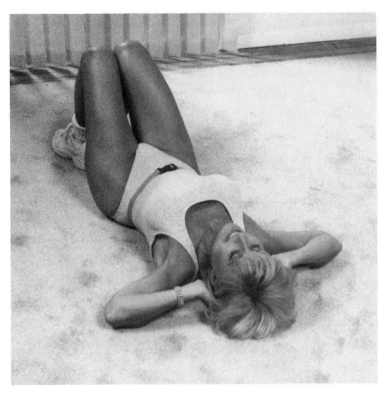

BACK PRESS KNEE RAISE: FINISH

Warm-Up #2: Dinosaur Curl

This exercise stretch relaxes and strengthens the abdominal and lower back areas.

POSITION

Lie on the floor and bend your knees, placing the soles of your feet flat on the floor. Cross your arms and hold either side of your front-side shoulder area. Make believe you are holding an orange between your chin and neck throughout the movement.

ACTION

Pretending that you are a dinosaur with each of your long vertebrae buried in the sand, slowly curl yourself up, beginning with your neck and moving your shoulders forward. Imagine each vertebra individually leaving the sand. You should move up until your head and shoulders are at an approximate 45-degree angle from the floor.

TIPS

Move very slowly. You should count to five on the way up, and five on the way down. You may repeat this stretch two more times.

Note: This is a modified version of Dr. Jack Barnathan's "Stegosaurus Sit-Up." He came up with the wonderful idea of imagining your vertebrae to be the spine of a "stegosaurus" dinosaur—with each vertebra buried in the sand.

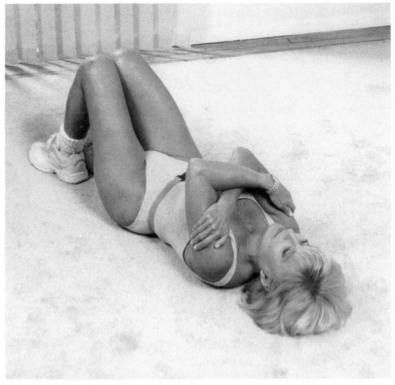

DINOSAUR CURL: START

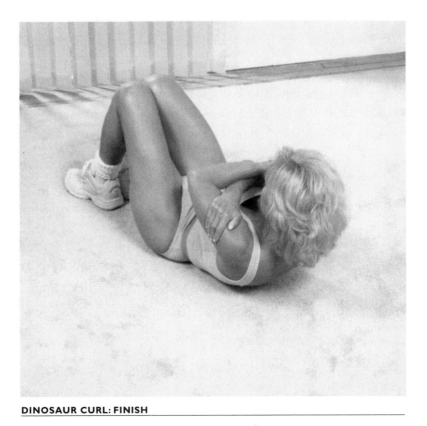

DINOSAUR CURL: FINISH

Exercise #1: Leaning One-Arm Dumbbell Row

This exercise develops, shapes, strengthens, and defines the entire latissimus dorsi muscle, strengthens the back muscles in general, and fortifies the spinal column. There is a side benefit to the arms.

POSITION

Bending at the waist, lean on a chair or exercise bench with one arm for support. Hold a dumbbell in your other hand, palm facing your body. Let your arm hang down until fully extended, allowing the weight of the dumbbell to stretch out your back muscles. Your back should be parallel to the floor, your shoulders evenly balanced, and your neck in line with your back.

ACTION

Keeping your working elbow close to your body at all times and flexing your back muscles, raise your elbow as high as possible. Return to start and feel the stretch in your back muscles. Repeat the movement until you have completed your set. Repeat for the other side of your back. Do your second and third sets.

TIPS

Go all the way up and all the way down for each movement. Keep your working elbow close to your body at all times. "Tell" your back and not your arms to do the work. Don't jerk the dumbbell up or nearly let it drop down.

MACHINES, ETC.

You can substitute this exercise by using any lat pulldown machine, doing the "lat pulldown to the front."

SETS, REPETITIONS, WEIGHTS

SET 1: 12 repetitions with lightest weight; rest for 15–30 seconds
SET 2: 10 repetitions with middle weight; rest for 15–30 seconds
SET 3: 8 repetitions with heaviest weight; rest for 15–30 seconds

REMINDER

See pages 55–57 for tips on heaviness of weights.

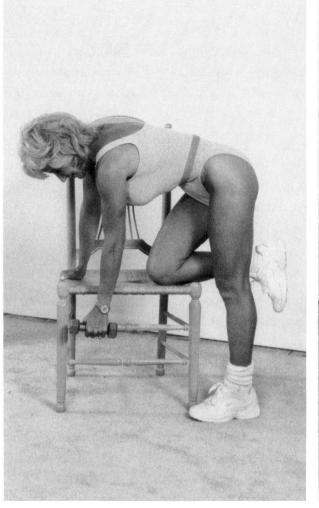

LEANING ONE-ARM DUMBBELL ROW: START

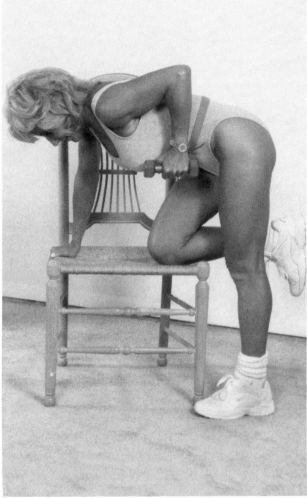

LEANING ONE-ARM DUMBBELL ROW: FINISH

Exercise #2: Back Overhead Pullover

This exercise develops, shapes, strengthens, and defines the upper back and latissimus dorsi muscle, and strengthens and builds the bones in the entire spinal column. It helps strengthen the back muscles in general. There is a side benefit to the chest.

POSITION

Lie on a flat exercise bench or "step" with knees bent and the soles of your feet flat on the floor. Press your back into the bench so there is no arching. Hold a dumbbell above your chest area with both hands, palms up, letting the dumbbell hang down between the triangle formed by your thumb and pointer fingers (see start photograph).

ACTION

In full control and bending at the elbows, lower your arms over your head and behind you until you feel a full stretch in your latissimus dorsi and upper back muscles. Flexing your latissimus dorsi and upper back muscles as you go, return to the start position. Repeat the movement until you have completed your set. Do your second and third sets.

TIPS

"Tell" your back muscles to do the work. Don't jerk the dumbbell up or nearly let it drop down. Keep your back flat on the bench. Don't hold your breath. Breathe naturally.

MACHINES, ETC.

You may substitute any back "pullover" machine for this exercise.

SETS, REPETITIONS, WEIGHTS

SET 1: 12 repetitions with lightest weight; rest for 15–30 seconds

SET 2: 10 repetitions with middle weight; rest for 15–30 seconds

SET 3: 8 repetitions with heaviest weight; rest for 15–30 seconds

REMINDER

See pages 55–57 for tips on heaviness of weights.

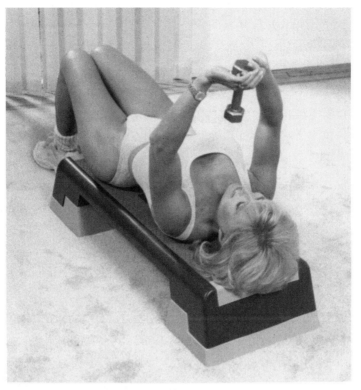

BACK OVERHEAD PULLOVER: START

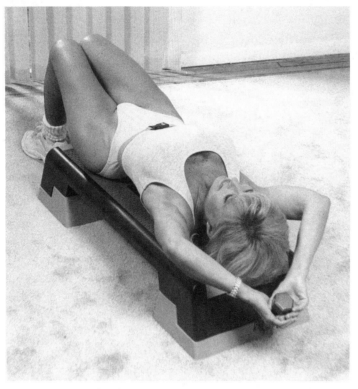

BACK OVERHEAD PULLOVER: FINISH

Exercise #3: Double-Arm Upright Row

This exercise develops, shapes, strengthens, and defines the entire trapezius muscle and strengthens and builds the bones in the entire spinal column. It also helps strengthen the shoulder joints. There is a side benefit to the biceps.

STANCE

Holding a dumbbell in each hand, palms facing your body, stand with your feet a natural width apart. Extend your arms fully downward, positioning each dumbbell in the center of each thigh.

ACTION

Flexing your trapezius muscles as you go and extending your elbows outward, and keeping the dumbbells close to your body, raise the dumbbells until they reach nearly chin height. In full control, return to start position. Feel the stretch in your trapezius, shoulder, and upper back muscles, and repeat the movement until you have completed your set. Do your second and third sets.

TIPS

Keep the dumbbells close to your body as you move. On the final up position, your elbows should be approximately shoulder height and parallel to the floor. Don't cheat the movement. Go all the way up and all the way down in full control. Don't hold your breath. Breathe naturally.

MACHINES, ETC.

You may do this exercise on any floor pulley machine.

SETS, REPETITIONS, WEIGHTS

SET 1: 12 repetitions with lightest weight; rest for 15–30 seconds

SET 2: 10 repetitions with middle weight; rest for 15–30 seconds

SET 3: 8 repetitions with heaviest weight; rest for 15–30 seconds

REMINDER

See pages 55–57 for tips on heaviness of weights.

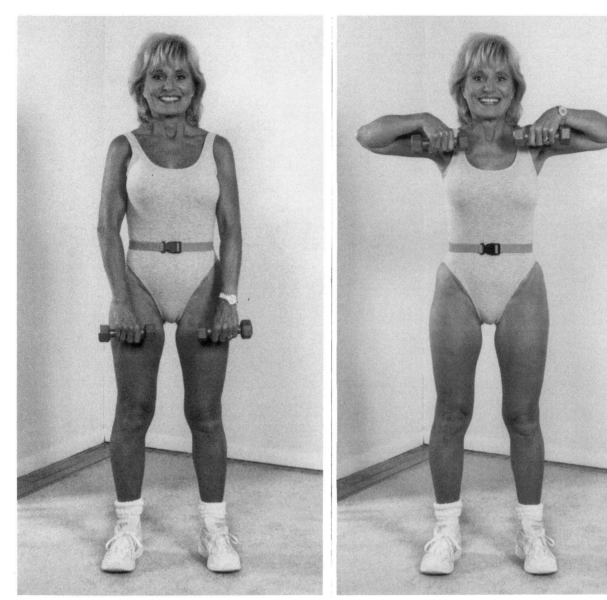

DOUBLE-ARM UPRIGHT ROW: START

DOUBLE-ARM UPRIGHT ROW: FINISH

Exercise #1: Crunch

This exercise develops, strengthens, and defines the upper abdominal muscles and helps strengthen the spinal column. There is a side benefit to the lower abdominals.

POSITION

Lie on a mat or rug on your back with your knees bent, and the soles of your feet on the floor. Place your hands behind your neck. (You will forget your arms. You will not use them to give you momentum.)

ACTION

Flexing your abdominal muscles as you go, in full control, raise your shoulders off the ground until you reach just under a 45-degree angle. In full control, return to the start position and repeat the movement until you have completed your set. Do your second and third sets.

TIPS

If you are sure you can resist pulling on your neck, extend your arms out at your sides. Don't jerk up and down or use your arms for momentum. Concentrate on your abdominal muscles as you work. Don't hold your breath. Breathe naturally.

MACHINES, ETC.

You may perform this exercise on any abdominal crunch machine.

SETS, REPETITIONS, WEIGHTS

SET 1: 15–25 repetitions with no weight; rest for 15–30 seconds
SET 2: 15–25 repetitions with no weight; rest for 15–30 seconds
SET 3: 15–25 repetitions with no weight; rest for 15–30 seconds

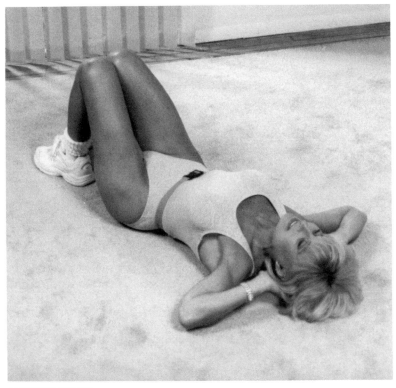

CRUNCH: START

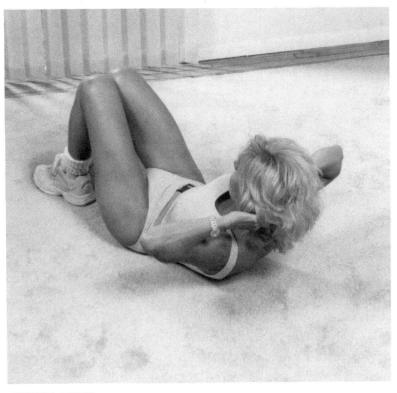

CRUNCH: FINISH

Exercise #2: Bent-Knee Sewn Lift

This exercise develops, strengthens, and defines the lower abdominal muscles and helps strengthen the spinal column. There is a side benefit to the lower back and upper abdominals.

POSITION

Lie on a mat or rug and bend at the knees. Place your hands behind your head. Press your back into the floor so that there is no arch whatsoever.

ACTION

Before you start moving, pretend that your belly button is sewn to the floor and keep this image in your mind the whole time. Now, flexing your lower abdominals as you go, slightly lift your hips toward the ceiling (about two to four inches), all the time keeping your back pressed to the floor. In full control and continuing to flex your lower abdominal muscles, return to the start position and repeat the movement until you have completed your set. Do your second and third sets.

TIPS

Resist jerking your hips up and nearly letting them drop down. Maintain full control at all times. Concentrate on flexing your abdominal muscles throughout the movement. At first this exercise seems tedious, but soon you'll learn to love it. Don't hold your breath. Breathe naturally.

MACHINES, ETC.

You may substitute any "lower abdominal" exercise done on an abdominal machine for this exercise.

SETS, REPETITIONS, WEIGHTS

SET 1: 15–25 repetitions with no weight; rest for 15–30 seconds

SET 2: 15–25 repetitions with no weight; rest for 15–30 seconds

SET 3: 15–25 repetitions with no weight; rest for 15–30 seconds

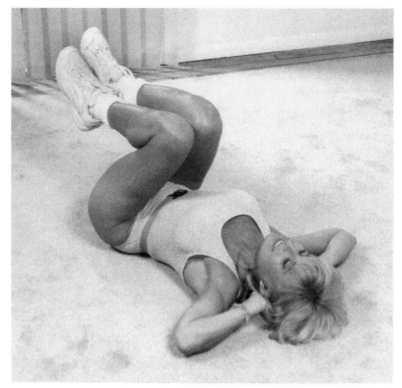

BENT-KNEE SEWN LIFT: START

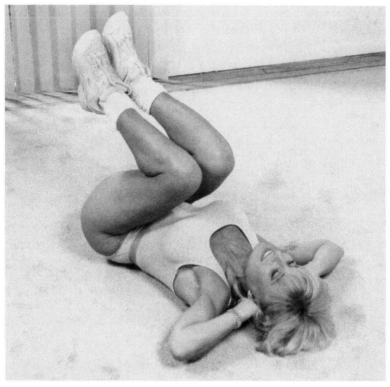

BENT-KNEE SEWN LIFT: FINISH

Exercise #3: Ceiling Lift

This exercise develops, strengthens, and defines the lower abdominal muscles and helps strengthen the spinal column. There is a side benefit to the lower back and upper abdominals.

POSITION

Lie on a mat or rug, placing your hands behind your neck. Raise your legs off the floor, extending your legs fully upward, with your knees bent very slightly and crossing your legs at the ankles. Press your back into the mat—no arching!

ACTION

Exactly as you did in exercise #2, before you begin, pretend your belly button is sewn to the floor. Keeping your legs extended upward the whole time and flexing your lower abdominals as you go, lift your hips toward the ceiling (about 2–4 inches), all the time keeping your back pressed to the floor. In full control and continuing to flex your lower abdominal muscles, return to the start position, and repeat the movement until you have completed your set. Do your second and third sets.

TIPS

This exercise is exactly the same as the bent-knee sewn lift, only this time your legs are extended upward, making the exercise a little more difficult. Don't cheat by letting your legs descend slowly. Remember to imagine that your belly button is sewn to the floor.

MACHINES, ETC.

You may substitute any "lower abdominal" exercise done on an abdominal machine for this exercise.

SETS, REPETITIONS, WEIGHTS

SET 1: 15–25 repetitions with no weight; rest for 15–30 seconds
SET 2: 15–25 repetitions with no weight; rest for 15–30 seconds
SET 3: 15–25 repetitions with no weight; rest for 15–30 seconds

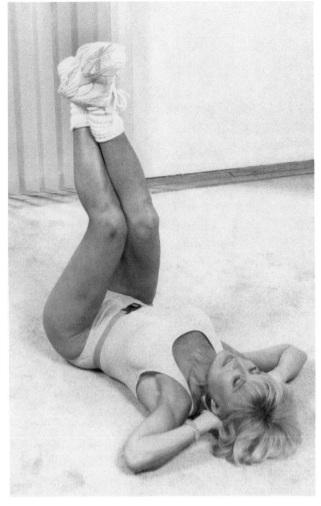

CEILING LIFT: START

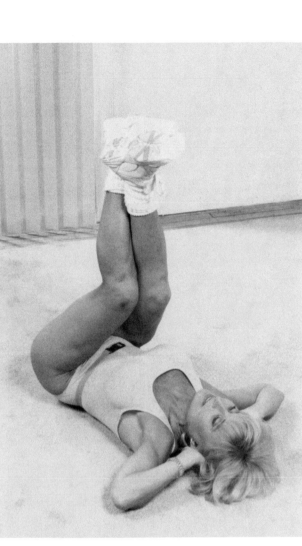

CEILING LIFT: FINISH

Review of Exercises in This Chapter

Back-Abdominal Workout

WARM-UPS: back press knee raise, dinosaur curl

BACK EXERCISES

1. Leaning one-arm dumbbell row
2. Back overhead pullover
3. Double-arm upright row

ABDOMINAL EXERCISES

1. Crunch
2. Bent-knee sewn lift
3. Ceiling lift

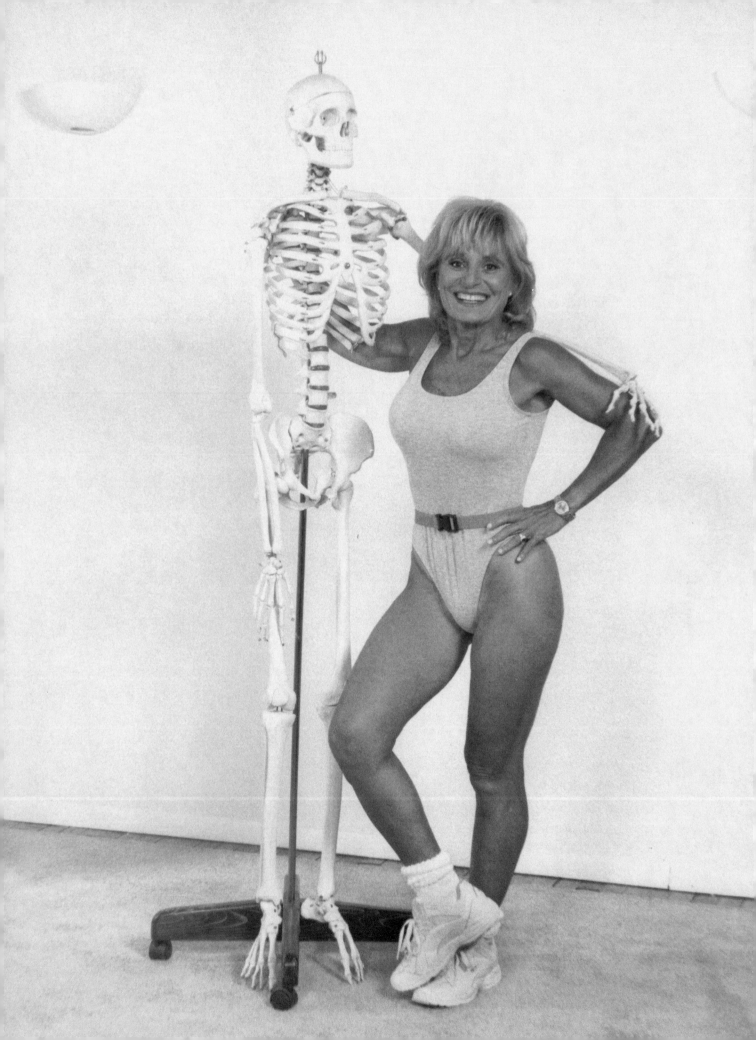

6. Leg and Hip/Buttocks for Muscle Tone, Beauty, Bone, and Strength

Why group the leg and hip/buttocks muscles together? They work in conjunction with each other and, in addition, when one is injured, the other is often affected. But more important, the exercises that help strengthen, shape, tighten, tone, and define the hip/buttocks muscles and strengthen the hip/buttocks area bones also have a positive effect on the legs. And the reverse is true about the leg workout.

The hip is one of the three most common fracture sites when bones are thinning (the spine and the wrist are the other two). A fractured hip can seriously impact quality of life because it often leads to the inability to walk. In fact, one-third of those who reach ninety will have fractured a hip! But, you may argue, "I'm far from ninety." Well, it can and does start happening even after forty. But bone in the bank will make sure it does not happen to you. And let's remember the additional result of this workout: tight, toned, shapely hips, buttocks, thighs, and calves!

The long thigh bone, the femur, is what has actually fractured when the doctor says you have fractured your hip. The most common fracture occurs at the upper end of the femur that connects to the hip, where the femur fits into a socket in the pelvis. This joint allows the hip to have circular motion. When bones are thinning, any slight impact or pressure on the upper thighbone where it is joined to the hip can cause a fracture in two areas: the neck of the femur and along the intertrochanteric line (an imaginary line connecting the two bony knobs on the upper femur that help to pull the hip muscles).

This chapter discusses exercising first your leg and then your hip/buttocks muscles and underlying bones. For a detailed description and anatomy photographs, see pages 38 and 39. Before beginning this workout, refer to the anatomy photograph and bone diagram, and locate the muscles and bones in your own body. This way, as you work out, you'll be able to "tell" your own muscles and bones to develop and strengthen. You can use your mind to help accelerate your progress.

The leg muscles targeted here are the **quadriceps,** located in the front thigh, originating at the hipbone and ending at the knee; the **sartoris,** which runs along the inner thigh from the hipbone to the inside of the knee; the **adductor,** which originates in the lower pelvic area on the pubis bone and rises to the shaft of the thighbone; the **biceps femoris,** or hamstrings, which originates in the bony area of the pelvis and terminates along the back of the knee joint; and the **gastrocnemius,** or calf muscle, which is located in the middle of the lower leg.

The leg bones that will be targeted are the **femur** (thighbone), which is attached to the pelvic girdle; the **patella** (kneecap), which is connected to the lower femur; the **tibia** (shinbone) and **fibula,** which run from the knee to the ankle and connect to the ankle bones **(tarsals).**

The hip/buttocks muscles targeted are the **gluteus maximus,** which begins at the thighbone and extends down the tailbone; the **gluteus medius,** which lies just beneath the gluteus maximus; and the **gluteus minimus,** which originates on the crest of the hipbone. The hip/buttocks bones targeted are the **pelvic bones,** which are composed of three bones: **ilium, ischium,** and **pubis.** These bones meet and form a cuplike socket called the **acetabulum,** to which the top of the femur (thighbone) is attached.

As you do your leg and hip/buttocks workout, remember to picture the muscles becoming tight and toned and strengthened, and envision the bones becoming denser. Also remember to be patient. The muscles of the legs and hip/buttocks may take a little longer than three weeks to show definite reshaping, but one thing is for sure: In a few months not only you but everyone will notice the difference in your muscles. And your bones, which nobody can see, will also be strengthening. That will be your hidden bonus—for life!

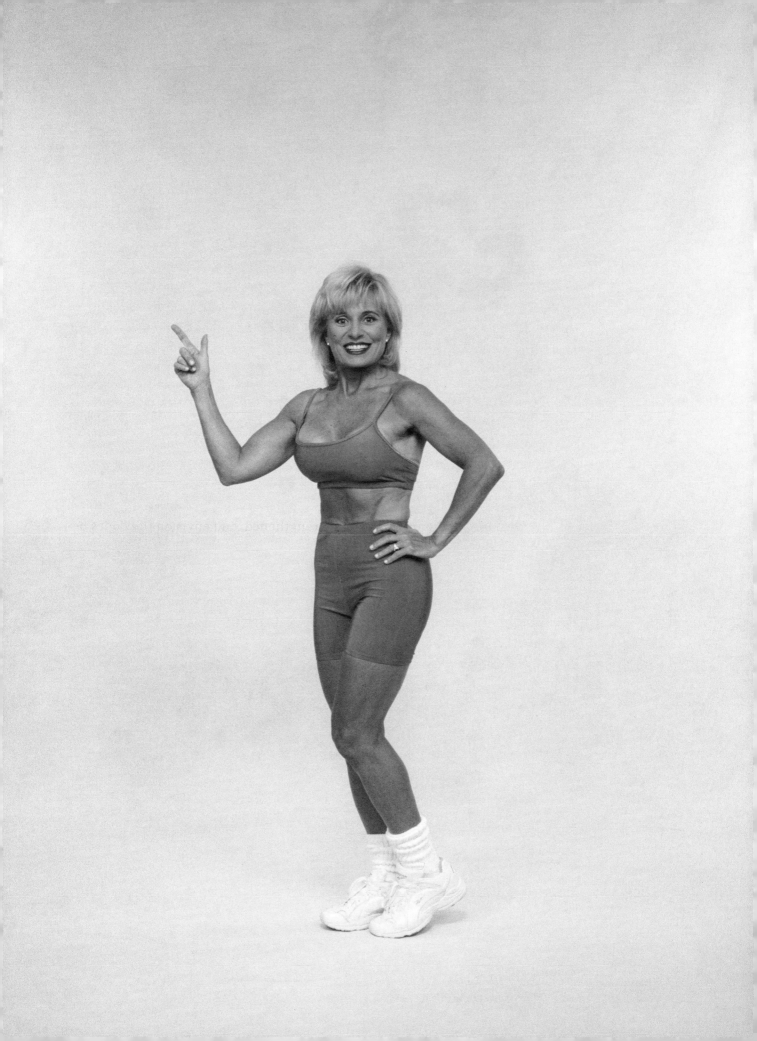

Warm-Up #1: Single Leg Extension

This exercise stretch relaxes and strengthens the muscles and bones in the entire front thigh area. There is a side benefit to the back thigh and the knee.

POSITION

With your knees about two inches apart, sit back in a chair that has a back. Place a folded towel under your knees so that your feet barely touch the floor. Your feet should be shoulder-width apart, and your hands should hold the sides of the chair or rest on your thighs.

ACTION

With your toes flexed toward your body and without using any weights, slowly extend one leg until your knee is nearly but not quite locked. Feel the stretch in your back thigh muscle. Slowly return to the start position and feel the stretch in your front thigh muscle. Repeat two more times and repeat for the other leg.

TIP

You may want to add to this stretch by circling your foot around to relax your ankle each time you return to the start position—before you perform your next repetition.

Note: This is an excellent exercise to use as a substitute for any leg exercise you can't do. In this case, you can use ankle weights, following the pyramid system described on page 28. (You would add a little weight to each set by slipping additional weight into the ankle weight slot for your second and third sets.) If you are substituting this and using it as an exercise, you will still do it as a stretch. Later, when you do it as an exercise, you will flex your front thigh muscle on the up movement for each repetition.

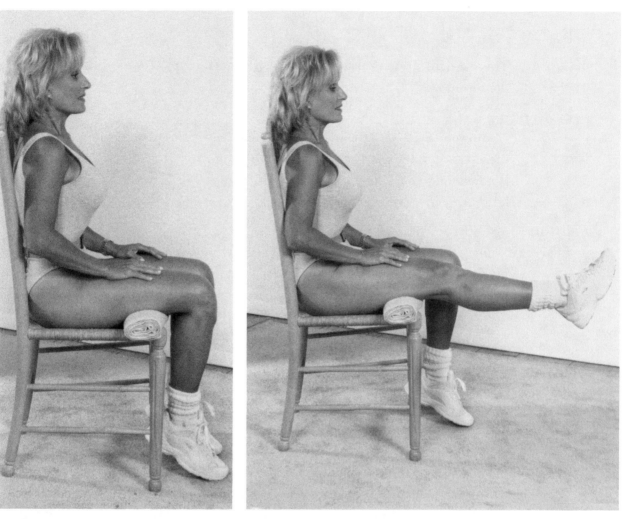

SINGLE LEG EXTENSION: START

SINGLE LEG EXTENSION: FINISH

Warm-Up #2: Lying Crossover

This exercise stretch relaxes and strengthens the hips. There is a side benefit to the lower back.

POSITION

Lie on your back with the soles of your feet flat on the floor. Press your back into the mat and interlock your fingers behind your head. Your arms should rest on the floor and your elbows should touch the floor. Cross your right leg over your left knee. (See start photograph.)

ACTION

Using your right leg to do the pulling, gently pull your left leg toward the floor, until you feel a nice stretch in your hip and lower back area, but go only as far as you can comfortably go without lifting your arms from the ground. (Don't dream that you will go all the way down to the floor. Most people go only a very short way.) Hold for ten seconds and repeat for the other leg. (Note: For this stretch, build up to twenty seconds on each side!)

TIPS

If you are really stiff and find that your arms leave the ground quite quickly, it's a good idea to do this stretch three times for each leg and to build up to twenty seconds. Be sure to keep your elbows and upper body as flat on the floor as possible throughout the stretch.

Note: I can only go a short way with this stretch, but it really makes my hip area feel relaxed. I used to hate this stretch, but now I love it.

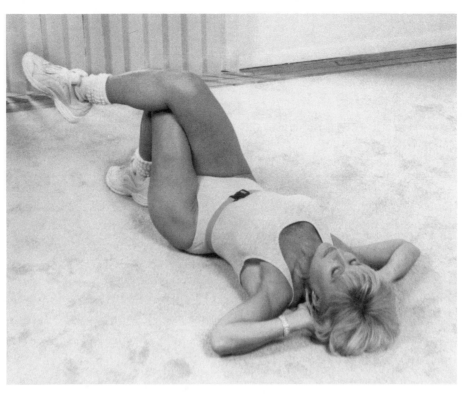

LYING CROSSOVER: START

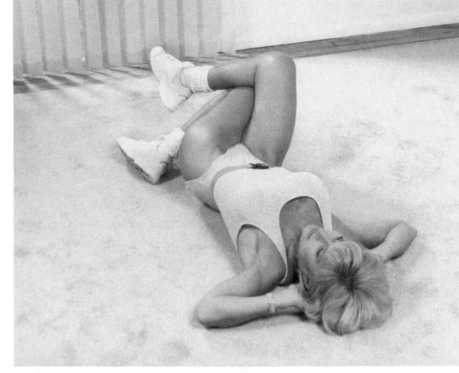

LYING CROSSOVER: FINISH

Exercise #1: Leg Curl

This exercise develops, shapes, and defines the back thigh muscle (hamstrings) and helps strengthen the knee (patella), thigh (femur), and shin (tibia and fibula) bones.

POSITION

Lie in a prone position on a mat or rug with your legs extended straight out and a dumbbell between your feet. Extend your arms out on the floor over your head.

ACTION

Bending your legs at the knees, raise them until they are perpendicular to the floor. Keep a firm grip on the dumbbell and flex your back thigh muscles as you go. In full control, return to the start position and repeat the movement until you have completed your set. Do your second and third sets.

TIPS

Wear sneakers and socks or your ankles will hurt! Feel your knees working as you go. Remember to feel the flex in your back thigh muscles on the up movement and the stretch on the down movement. Maintain control at all times. Don't start jerking the dumbbell up and nearly letting it drop down. You may replace the dumbbell with ankle weights, but the dumbbell is more effective because its placement forces the work to be done by the targeted muscles and bones.

MACHINES, ETC.

You may perform this exercise on any leg curl machine.

SETS, REPETITIONS, WEIGHTS

SET 1: 12 repetitions with lightest weight; rest for 15–30 seconds
SET 2: 10 repetitions with middle weight; rest for 15–30 seconds
SET 3: 8 repetitions with heaviest weight; rest for 15–30 seconds

REMINDER

See pages 55–57 for tips on heaviness of weights.

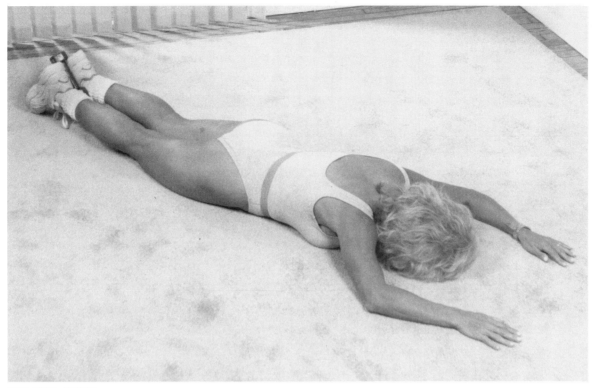

LEG CURL: START

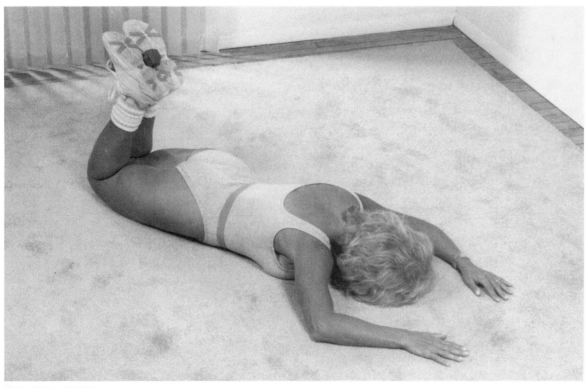

LEG CURL: FINISH

Exercise #2: Lunge

This exercise develops, shapes, strengthens, and defines the entire front thigh (quadriceps) muscle and strengthens the thigh, knee, and ankle bones. There is a side benefit to the inner and outer thigh muscles, the buttocks, and the hipbones.

STANCE

Stand with a dumbbell in each hand, palms facing your body, arms straight down at your sides, feet a natural width apart. Keep your back straight and look directly ahead of you.

ACTION

Keep your knee aligned with your toe and your nonstepping leg straight. Bending at the knee, step forward with one foot until you can just about see your toes. (If you cannot see your toes, you have stepped too far.) Feel the stretch in your stepping front thigh muscle and the flex in your nonstepping front thigh muscle. In full control and using the muscles in your lunging leg, not your back leg, return to the start position and repeat the movement for the other leg. Repeat the alternate lunging movement until you have completed your set. Do your second and third sets.

TIPS

Make sure that your working knee is not extended over your toes. Don't worry if you are awkward at first; in time you will gain balance. As you lunge forward, imagine that you are carrying a toolbox in each hand and, stepping forward, that you are lowering yourself to the ground to place the toolboxes down. This may help with balance. If you cannot lunge, you may substitute this exercise for the leg extension stretch exercise, using ankle weights.

MACHINES, ETC.

You may do leg presses on any leg press machine in place of this exercise.

SETS, REPETITIONS, WEIGHTS

SET 1: 12 repetitions with lightest weight; rest for 15–30 seconds
SET 2: 10 repetitions with middle weight; rest for 15–30 seconds
SET 3: 8 repetitions with heaviest weight; rest for 15–30 seconds

REMINDER

See pages 55–57 for tips on heaviness of weights.

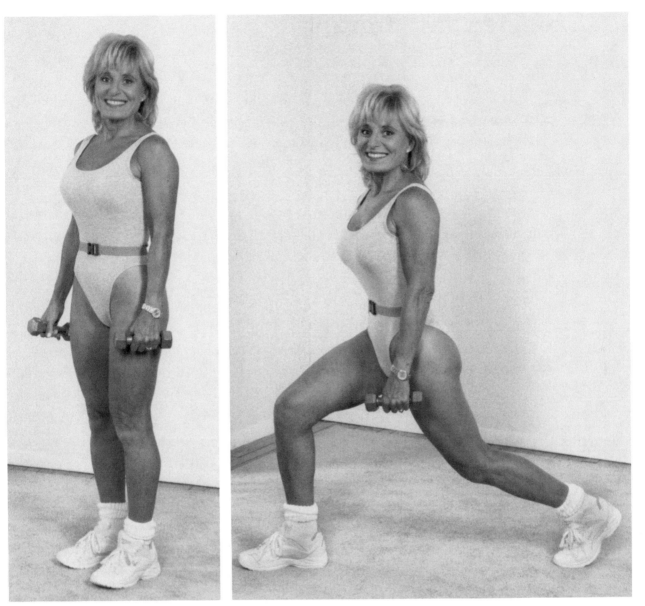

LUNGE: START

LUNGE: FINISH

Exercise #3: Inner Thigh Sweep

This exercise tightens, tones, and strengthens the inner thigh (adductor and sartoris) muscles and helps strengthen the hip joints and thighbone (femur). There is a side benefit to the muscles of the front and back thigh, and the hip/buttocks area.

STANCE

Stand near a chair for balance, with your feet shoulder-width apart. Place one hand on the top of the chair. (The seat of the chair is facing away from you so it is not in the way.) The leg closest to the chair remains stable throughout the set.

ACTION

Flexing your inner thigh muscles as you go, and pointing your foot slightly upward, making your heel brush the ground, "sweep" your leg forward in a diagonal motion until your heel passes the toes of your stable leg by an inch or two. In full control, return to the start position, feeling the stretch in your inner thigh muscles. Repeat the movement until you have completed your set. Perform the set for your other leg. Do your second and third sets.

TIPS

Keep your working knee nearly locked throughout the movement. Notice that when you point your toes slightly up as you move, letting your heel nearly brush the ground, you can really flex that inner thigh muscle! Don't bend over as you work. Stand upright! You will do this exercise without weights! You will be doing all the work yourself by consciously flexing on the sweep movement as hard as possible. Don't worry. In time you'll flex harder and harder—as your muscle gets stronger.

Note: If this exercise is too easy for you, and you feel you can do it, replace this exercise with the wide leg semi-squat (3a) or better, do it in addition to this one!

MACHINES, ETC.

You may substitute this exercise by using the hip adductor machine.

SETS, REPETITIONS, WEIGHTS

SET 1: 15–25 repetitions with no weight; rest for 15–30 seconds
SET 2: 15–25 repetitions with no weight; rest for 15–30 seconds
SET 3: 15–25 repetitions with no weight; rest for 15–30 seconds

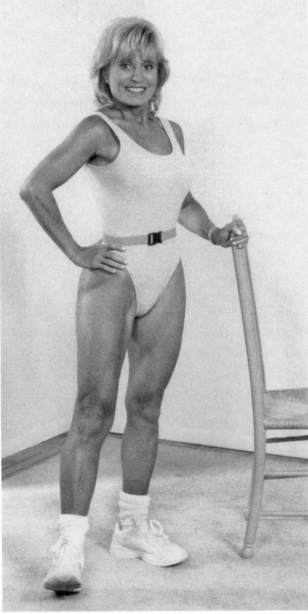

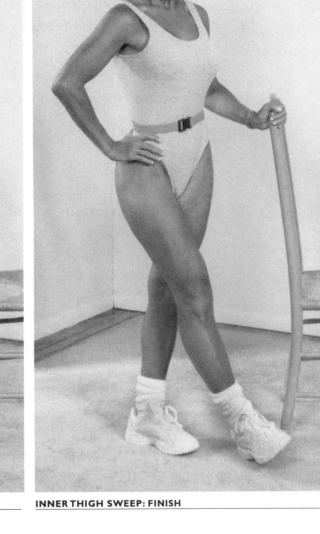

INNER THIGH SWEEP: START

INNER THIGH SWEEP: FINISH

Exercise 3a: Wide Leg Semi-Squat

This exercise develops, shapes, strengthens, and defines the front thigh (quadriceps) and inner thigh (adductor and sartoris) muscles and strengthens the hip joints and thighbone (femur). There is a side benefit to the hip/buttocks area, shinbones, and spinal column.

STANCE

Hold a dumbbell in the center of your body, palms facing your body, and stand with your feet very wide apart—about three to five inches wider than shoulder width. Your toes should be pointed outward. Your arms are straight down in front of you. Keep your back straight and look straight ahead.

ACTION

Feeling the stretch in your front thigh muscles as you go, descend to a bend in your knees of approximately 45 degrees. But don't go that low if you feel a strain in your knees. Flexing your front thigh muscles as you go and leading with your chest and chin, return to the start position. Give your front thigh muscles an extra "flex" and repeat the movement until you have completed your set. Do your second and third sets.

TIPS

This is a "semi-squat," so go only as far as is comfortable for you. If you find your heels rising off the ground, your feet are not wide enough.

MACHINES, ETC.

You may do this exercise on any squat machine.

SETS, REPETITIONS, WEIGHTS

SET 1: 12 repetitions with lightest weight; rest for 15–30 seconds
SET 2: 10 repetitions with middle weight; rest for 15–30 seconds
SET 3: 8 repetitions with heaviest weight; rest for 15–30 seconds

REMINDER

See pages 55–57 for tips on heaviness of weights.

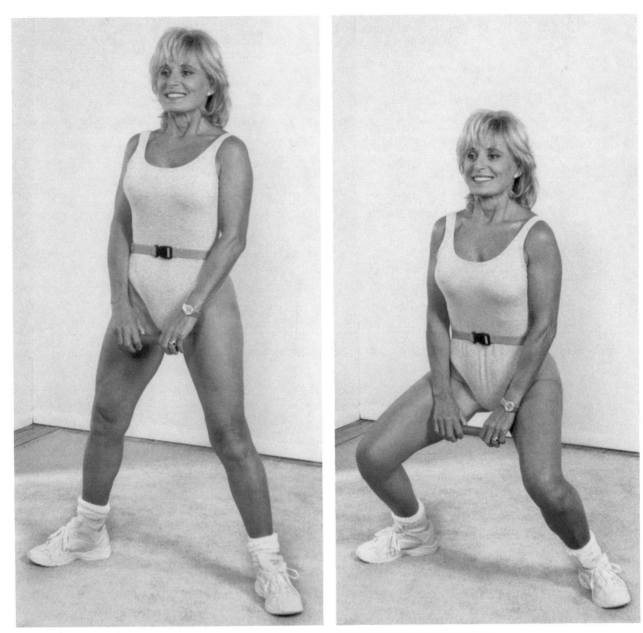

WIDE LEG SEMI-SQUAT: START

WIDE LEG SEMI-SQUAT: FINISH

Exercise #4: Standing Calf Raise

This exercise develops, shapes, strengthens, and defines the calf (gastrocnemius and soleus) muscles and helps strengthen the ankle bones. There is a side benefit to the shin and thigh bones.

STANCE

Stand by a chair with its back facing you. Your feet should be about a foot apart, toes pointed slightly outward.

ACTION

Using the back of the chair for balance if you need it, and flexing your calf muscles as you go, rise up on the toes of your feet as high as possible. Give your calf muscles an extra flex and, feeling the stretch in your calf muscles, return to the start position. Without bouncing and in full control, repeat the movement until you have completed your set. Do your second and third sets.

TIPS

You don't need weight for this exercise because your entire body serves as "the weight." If your calf muscles and ankles are weak, you may not be able to lift yourself all the way up at first. Don't worry. In time you will get stronger. If you are using the chair for balance, merely let your fingertips graze the chair—don't lean on it. Later you can do one leg at a time for even more effect!

MACHINES, ETC.

You may do this exercise on any standing calf machine.

SETS, REPETITIONS, WEIGHTS

SET 1: 15–25 repetitions with no weight; rest for 15–30 seconds

SET 2: 15–25 repetitions with no weight; rest for 15–30 seconds

SET 3: 15–25 repetitions with no weight; rest for 15–30 seconds

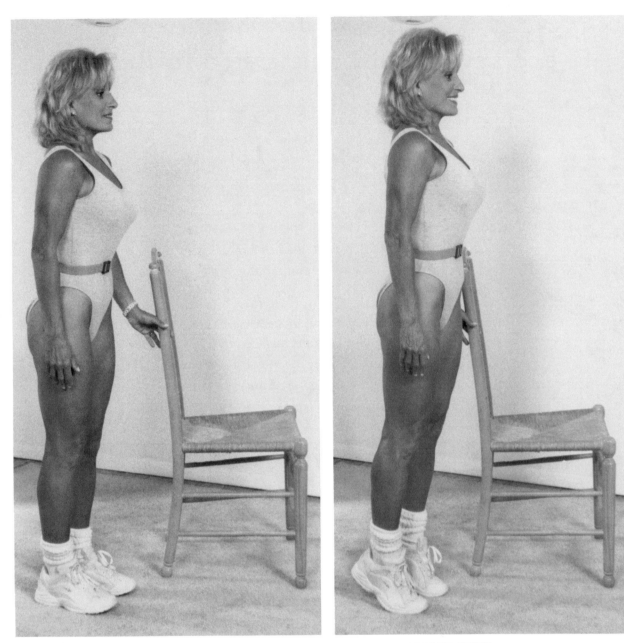

STANDING CALF RAISE: START

STANDING CALF RAISE: FINISH

Exercise #1: Alternate Prone Butt Lift

This exercise tightens, tones, shapes, and defines the entire hip/buttocks area and helps strengthen the bones in the hip and pelvic areas. There is a side benefit to the front and back thighs.

POSITION

Lie on a mat or rug facedown on the floor, your arms extended straight out in front of you or with your hands folded in front of your head, or you may rest on your elbows. Your toes should be pointed down and your feet about a foot apart.

ACTION

Working one buttock at a time and flexing as you go, without bending your knee, lift one leg until you cannot comfortably go any higher. Continuing to flex your working buttock muscle and in full control, return to the start position and repeat the movement for the other leg. Continue this alternate movement until you have completed your set. Do your second and third sets.

TIPS

Keep your back relaxed as you work. Don't arch it. Don't hold your breath. Breathe naturally.

MACHINES, ETC.

You may substitute this exercise for any exercise performed on a hip/buttocks machine.

SETS, REPETITIONS, WEIGHTS

SET 1: 15–25 repetitions with no weight; rest for 15–30 seconds

SET 2: 15–25 repetitions with no weight; rest for 15–30 seconds

SET 3: 15–25 repetitions with no weight; rest for 15–30 seconds

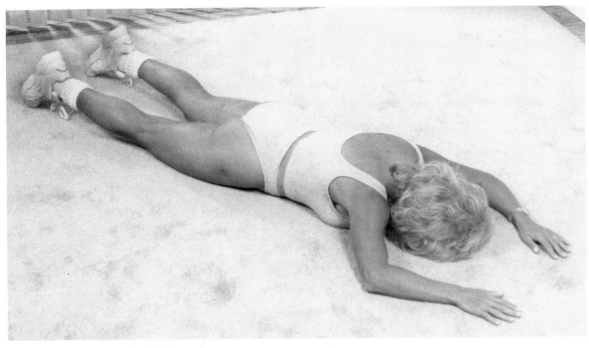

ALTERNATE PRONE BUTT LIFT: START

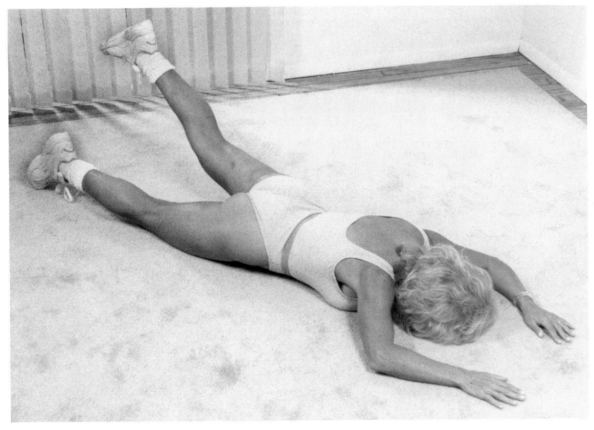

ALTERNATE PRONE BUTT LIFT: FINISH

Exercise #2: Lying Butt Lift

This exercise tightens, tones, shapes, and defines the entire hip/buttocks area and helps strengthen the bones in the hip and pelvic areas. There is a side benefit to the abdominal and lower back areas.

POSITION

Lie on a mat or rug, pressing your back into the mat. Place the soles of your feet flat on the floor. With your arms at your sides, place the palms of your hands on the floor, or fold your hands behind your head.

ACTION

Flexing your entire hip/buttocks area as you go, raise your hips slightly off the floor by pressing your back even further into the mat. You will be raising your hips by about three inches. In full control, return to the start position and repeat the movement until you have completed your set. Do your second and third sets.

TIPS

Be sure to keep a full flex on your hip/buttocks muscles on the up movement and momentarily relax on the down movement. Don't jerk up and down. The key to this exercise is concentration and control. Don't hold your breath. Breathe naturally.

MACHINES, ETC.

You may substitute this exercise for any exercise done on a hip/buttocks machine.

SETS, REPETITIONS, WEIGHTS

SET 1: 15–25 repetitions with no weight; rest for 15–30 seconds
SET 2: 15–25 repetitions with no weight; rest for 15–30 seconds
SET 3: 15–25 repetitions with no weight; rest for 15–30 seconds

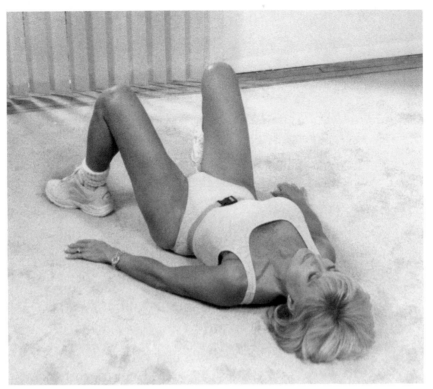

LYING BUTT LIFT: START

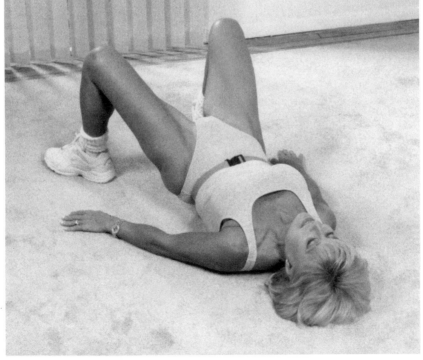

LYING BUTT LIFT: FINISH

Leg and Hip/Buttocks for Muscle Tone, Beauty, Bone, and Strength   107

Exercise #3:
Standing Bent-Knee Back Leg Extension

This exercise tightens, tones, shapes, and defines the entire hip/buttocks, especially the "saddlebags" area, and helps strengthen the bones in the hip and pelvic regions. There is a side benefit to the knees and the front and back thighs.

STANCE

Standing near a chair, gently hold the back of the chair with one hand for balance. Your back should be straight and your feet shoulder-width apart. Bend your working leg at the knee.

ACTION

Flexing your working hip/buttocks muscle as you go, extend your leg diagonally out behind you and stop just short of locking your knee. Return to start position and repeat the movement until you have completed your set. Repeat the movement with the other leg. Do your second and third sets.

TIPS

You may place your hand on your working buttock to feel yourself flexing your buttock. This will encourage you to flex harder and get more out of the exercise. Don't hold your breath. Breathe naturally.

MACHINES, ETC.

You may substitute this exercise for any exercise performed on a hip/buttocks machine.

SETS, REPETITIONS, WEIGHTS

SET 1: 15–25 repetitions with no weight; rest for 15–30 seconds

SET 2: 15–25 repetitions with no weight; rest for 15–30 seconds

SET 3: 15–25 repetitions with no weight; rest for 15–30 seconds

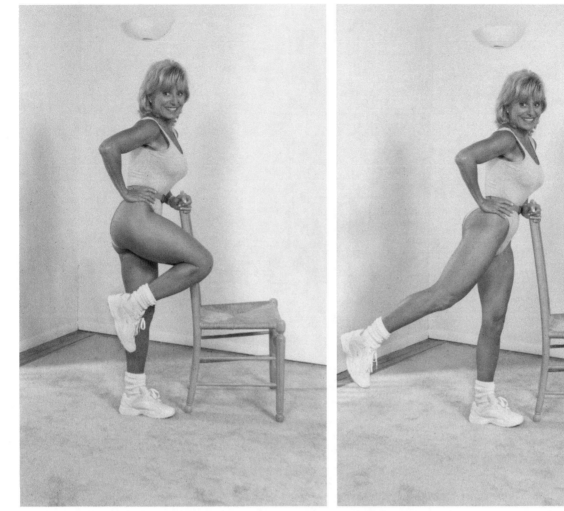

STANDING BENT-KNEE BACK LEG EXTENSION: START

STANDING BENT-KNEE BACK LEG EXTENSION: FINISH

Review of Exercises in This Chapter

Leg-Hip/Buttocks Workout

WARM-UPS: single leg extension, lying crossover

LEG EXERCISES

    1. Leg curl

    2. Lunge

    3. Inner thigh sweep or

    3a. Wide leg semi-squat

    4. Standing calf raise

HIP/BUTTOCKS EXERCISES

    1. Alternate prone butt lift

    2. Lying butt lift

    3. Standing bent-knee back leg extension

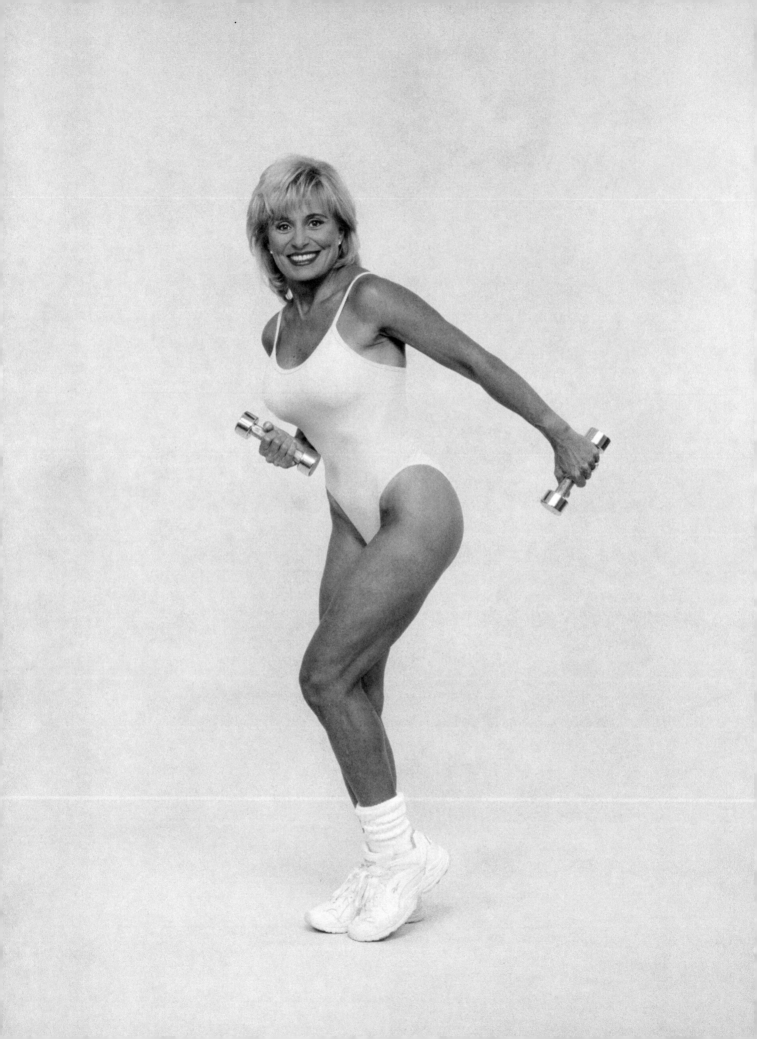

7. Arms: Wrist, Biceps, and Triceps for Muscle Tone, Beauty, Bone, and Strength

Let's think about the arms. We use them for everything: carrying things, pushing doors open, holding weights to do exercises, hugging loved ones, and even to express ourselves (gesturing while conversing, such as tapping our forehead to express "oh, no!"). Simply put, we need strong muscles and bones in our arms for everyday living. But the arms also tell a lot about the shape we are in!

Many women forget this fact. They become so involved with shaping up the thighs, hips, butt, and stomach that they forget the body part which is almost impossible to hide, especially in hot weather. So why not gain the beautiful arms that will come with the arm workout—the pretty, well-shaped biceps muscle and a tight-toned triceps muscle (the area of your arm located between the elbow and armpit, the one that "waves like a flag" when you raise your arm after a certain age, if you're badly out of shape).

One part of the arm, the wrist, is one of the three most common bone fracture sites. (The spine and the hips are the other two.) This is so because when you fall (and most of us do at one time or another), the first thing you do is stretch out your hands to break the fall. If your wrist bone (radius) is weak, you fracture it, usually on the joint surface where it connects to the forearm. There are many types of wrist fractures including those where the wrist bone breaks but remains in place and the more complex fractures where the wrist bone is broken in a few different directions, especially toward the back of the forearm (Colles' fracture). Your first two exercises in this workout will focus on the wrist area, but all the exercises you do using dumbbells will help strengthen your wrists.

It's quite wonderful that we now know that by doing specific weight-training exercises, we can not only reshape the muscles and gain firm, shapely arms but also strengthen the underlying bone so that we can enjoy our sports, adventures, and daily activities with ease, no matter what our age. In this chapter you'll be exercising your wrists and forearms first. Then you'll move to your biceps and triceps. In the end you will have thoroughly covered your entire arm.

The wrist muscles we'll be targeting here are the **flexor carpi radialis, flexor carpi ulnaris, extensor carpi radialis longus,** and **extensor carpi radialis brevis,** which run up through the forearms, and the **brachioradialis**—a muscle that originates at the end of the humerus bone and is attached to the surface of the **radius.** (Technically speaking, the muscles of the forearm are considered wrist muscles.)

The wrist bones that concern us here are located at the end of the forearm—the radius on the inner side of the arm (vertical to the thumb) and the **ulna** on the outer side of the arm (vertical to the pinkie finger). Both bones are attached to the upper arm bone, the **humerus,** and are connected at the elbow joint. The lower part of the ulna forms a major part of the wrist, which is why the technical word for wrist is "ulna."

The biceps and triceps muscles are undergirded by common bones, so we'll discuss them together. The **biceps** begins at the shoulder blade and ends at the forearm. The **triceps** originates at the shoulder blade and the upper arm, and inserts at the elbow. The upper arm bone that concerns us is the long, strong humerus, which is located under the biceps and triceps muscles.

As you do your arm exercises, remember to envision the muscles becoming tight and toned and shapely, and to imagine the bones strengthening. The good news about the arms is that they show some outward improvement within three to four weeks!

Note: You will perform two quick warm-up stretches for the arms. One is for the wrist and forearm, the other is for the biceps and triceps.

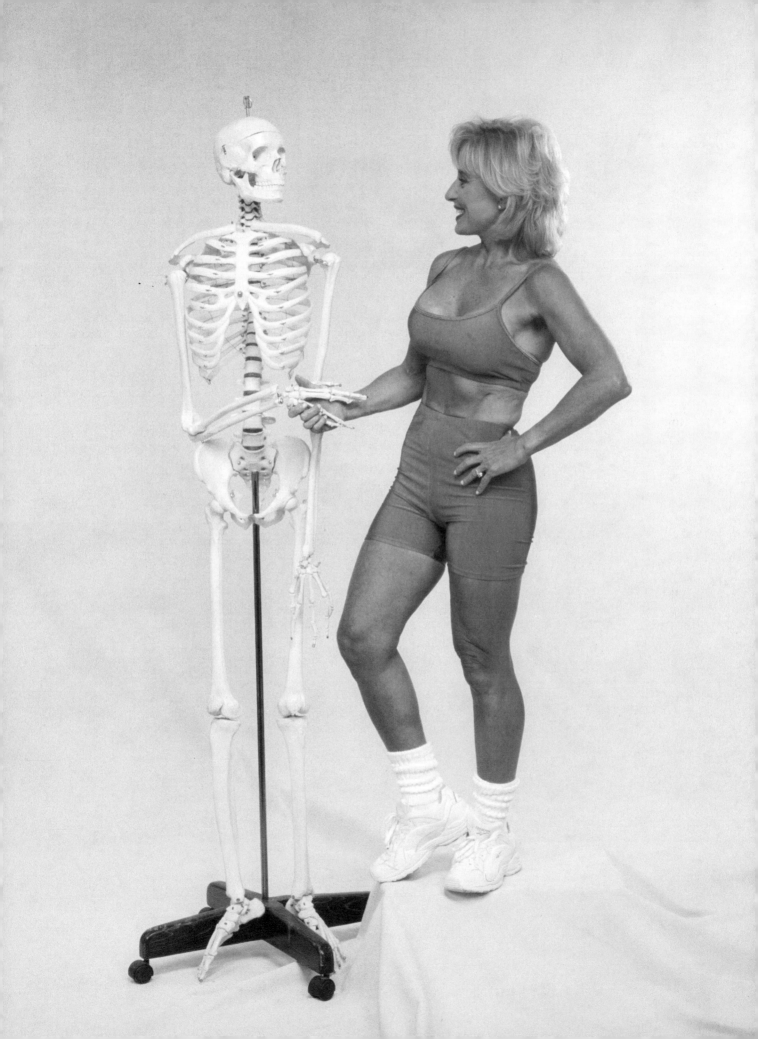

Warm-Up #1:
Doggie Paw Wrist-Forearm Stretch

This exercise stretch relaxes and strengthens the entire forearm and wrist areas and will help you do the palms-up wrist curl and the palms-down wrist raise with ease.

POSITION

Get into an "all fours" position, supporting yourself on your hands and knees, but instead of putting your hands in a normal position, reverse your hands by pointing your fingers toward your knees and your thumbs away from your body.

ACTION

Keeping the palms of your hands flat at all times, very gently lean back until you can feel a good stretch in your wrists and forearms. Hold for ten seconds, then return to the start position. Optional: repeat two more times.

TIPS

Don't push it. Just stretch enough to feel a gentle stretch. Don't be surprised if you feel very stiff in the wrist area. You will loosen up after a few weeks.

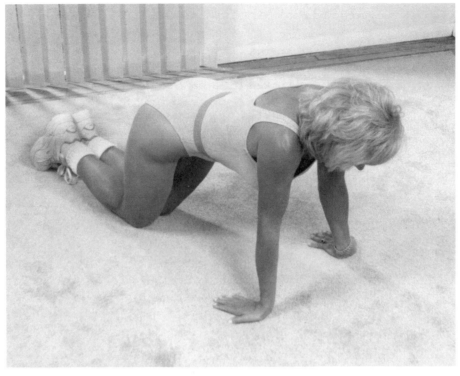

DOGGIE PAW WRIST-FOREARM STRETCH: START

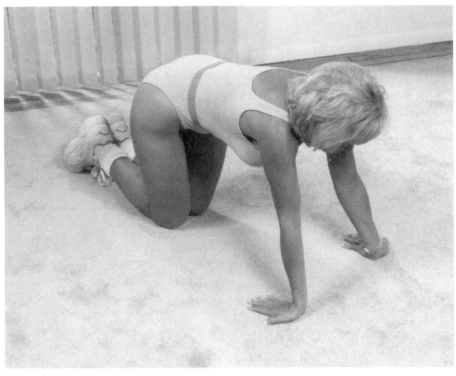

DOGGIE PAW WRIST-FOREARM STRETCH: FINISH

Arms: Wrist, Biceps, and Triceps for Muscle Tone, Beauty, Bone, and Strength   115

Warm-Up #2:
Scratch-Your-Back Biceps-Triceps Pull

This exercise stretch relaxes and loosens the entire biceps-triceps area and will help you perform your biceps and triceps exercises with greater ease. There is a side benefit to the trapezius and shoulder areas.

STANCE

Stand with your arms overhead and grip the elbow of one arm with the opposite hand. Let the elbow-gripped arm descend behind your back in a relaxed manner. (Your position will look as if you were going to scratch your back. See photograph.)

ACTION

Pull down on your elbow very gently in a behind-your-head direction until you feel a relaxing stretch. Hold for ten seconds. Repeat with the other arm. Optional: repeat two more times.

TIPS

Don't jerk your elbow down. Pull gently until you feel an easy stretch. Don't hold your breath. Breathe naturally. Since this is such an easy stretch, I find myself doing it during the day just to relax my shoulder and arm muscles.

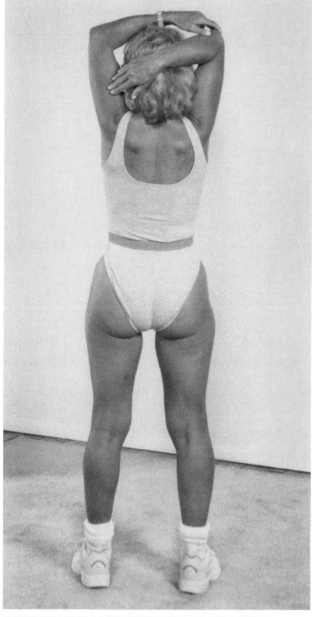

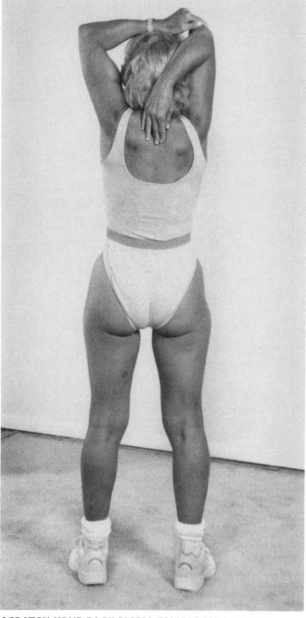

SCRATCH-YOUR-BACK BICEPS-TRICEPS PULL: START

SCRATCH-YOUR-BACK BICEPS-TRICEPS PULL: FINISH

Exercise #1: Palms-Up Wrist Curl

This exercise develops and shapes the forearm muscle, and strengthens and builds the wrist and forearm bones. There is a side benefit to the hand and finger bones (carpals, metacarpals, and phalanges).

POSITION

Keeping your feet flat on the floor, place yourself at the edge of an exercise bench or chair. Holding the dumbbells in each hand with palms facing up, lean forward and rest your forearms on your thighs. Relax your wrists downward with the dumbbell.

ACTION

Flexing your forearms as you go, curl your wrists upward as far as you can. Hold for a second and, without straining and in full control, return to the start position. Feel a full stretch in your wrist-forearm area and repeat the movement until you have completed your set. Do your second and third sets.

TIPS

Don't jerk the dumbbells up and let them drop down. Maintain control. Don't hold your breath. Breathe naturally. Let your mind cooperate with the movement. Mentally "tell" your wrist and forearm bones and muscles to grow stronger and more solid. You may do this exercise one arm at a time.

MACHINES, ETC.

You may perform this exercise with a light barbell.

SETS, REPETITIONS, WEIGHTS

SET 1: 12 repetitions with lightest weight; rest for 15–30 seconds

SET 2: 10 repetitions with middle weight; rest for 15–30 seconds

SET 3: 8 repetitions with heaviest weight; rest for 15–30 seconds

REMINDER

See pages 55–57 for tips on heaviness of weights and raising weights.

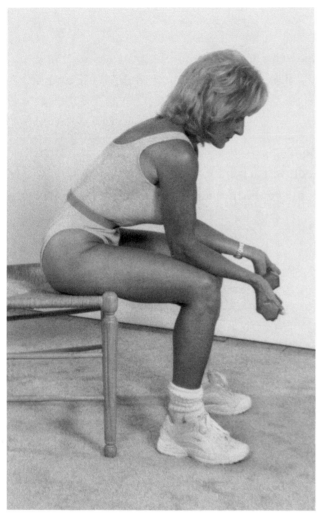 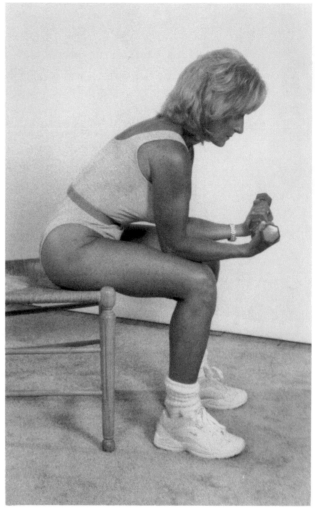

PALMS-UP WRIST CURL: START

PALMS-UP WRIST CURL: FINISH

Exercise #2: Palms-Down Wrist Raise

This exercise develops and shapes the forearm muscle, and strengthens and builds the wrist and forearm bones. There is a side benefit to the hand and finger bones.

POSITION

Keeping your feet flat on the floor, place yourself at the edge of an exercise bench or chair. Holding a dumbbell in each hand with palms facing down, lean forward and rest your forearms on your thighs. Relax your wrists downward with the dumbbell.

ACTION

Stretching your forearms as you go, flex your wrists upward as far as you can without straining and, in full control, hold for a second. Flexing your forearms as you go, return to the start position. Feel the stretch in your wrist area. Repeat the movement until you have completed your set. Do your second and third sets.

TIPS

Don't jerk the dumbbells up and let them drop down. Maintain control. Don't hold your breath. Breathe naturally. This wrist exercise is more challenging than the first. If you can't do it, wait until the first exercise (palms up) strengthens your wrist enough to do this one.

MACHINES, ETC.

You may perform this exercise with a light barbell.

SETS, REPETITIONS, WEIGHTS

SET 1: 12 repetitions with lightest weight; rest for 15–30 seconds

SET 2: 10 repetitions with middle weight; rest for 15–30 seconds

SET 3: 8 repetitions with heaviest weight; rest for 15–30 seconds

REMINDER

See pages 55–57 for tips on heaviness of weights and raising weights.

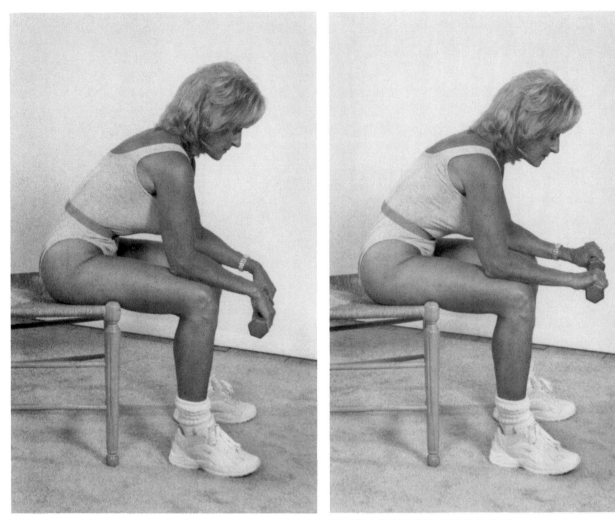

PALMS-DOWN WRIST RAISE: START

PALMS-DOWN WRIST RAISE: FINISH

Exercise #3:
Standing Simultaneous Curl

This exercise develops, shapes, and defines the entire biceps muscle and strengthens the underlying bone (humerus) and the wrist bones. There is a side benefit to the forearm and musculature of the entire upper arm.

STANCE

Stand with your feet a natural width apart and your knees very slightly bent. Hold a dumbbell in each hand, palms facing your body. Your arms should be straight down at your sides and close to your body.

ACTION

Flexing your biceps muscles as you go, curl your wrists to the front of your body. Bending at the elbows, curl your arms upward toward your shoulders until the dumbbells are about shoulder height. Without resting, return to the start position. Repeat the movement until you have completed your set. Do your second and third sets.

TIPS

Don't rock back and forth as you work the dumbbells. Keep a steady stance. Your palms should face your body at each return to start, and as you move the dumbbells up, curl your palms outward. (See photographs.)

MACHINES, ETC.

You may perform this exercise on any biceps curl machine.

SETS, REPETITIONS, WEIGHTS

SET 1: 12 repetitions with lightest weight; rest for 15–30 seconds

SET 2: 10 repetitions with middle weight; rest for 15–30 seconds

SET 3: 8 repetitions with heaviest weight; rest for 15–30 seconds

REMINDER

See pages 55–57 for tips on heaviness of weights.

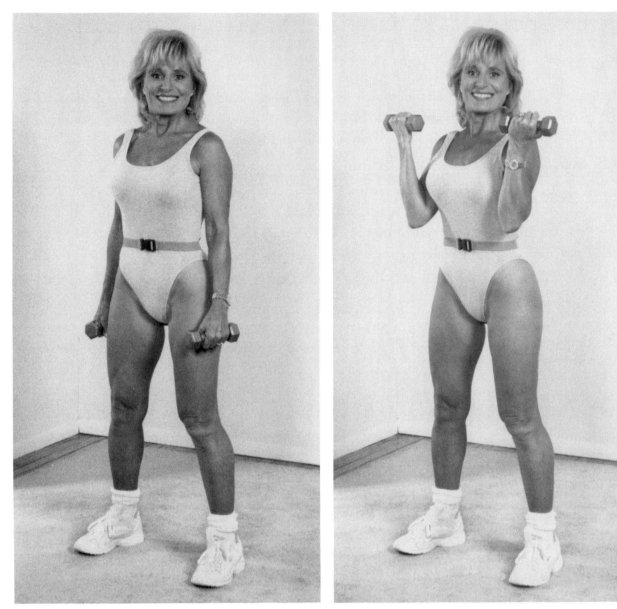

STANDING SIMULTANEOUS CURL: START

STANDING SIMULTANEOUS CURL: FINISH

Exercise #4: Concentration Curl

This exercise strengthens, develops, shapes, and defines the entire biceps muscle and strengthens the underlying bone (humerus). There is a side benefit to the wrist, forearm, and triceps muscles and bones.

POSITION

Holding a dumbbell in your right hand, palm away from your body, sit at the edge of a chair or an exercise bench and lean forward. Place your right elbow against your right inner thigh. Extend your arm fully downward and feel a full stretch in your biceps muscle. Keep your wrist very slightly curled upward. Place your other hand on your left thigh to support yourself.

ACTION

Flexing your biceps muscle as you go, curl your right arm upward toward your face as far as you can go (approximately chin height). Give your biceps muscle an extra flex and return to the start position, feeling your biceps muscle stretch out. Repeat the movement until you have completed your set. Repeat the set for your other arm. Do your second and third sets.

TIPS

Try to keep your head down throughout the movement. Make believe you are going to punch yourself in the face with the dumbbell each time. Don't swing the dumbbell up and down. Keep your wrist slightly curled throughout the movement. Maintain control at all times. Don't hold your breath. Breathe naturally.

MACHINES, ETC.

There is no machine substitute for this exercise.

SETS, REPETITIONS, WEIGHTS

SET 1: 12 repetitions with lightest weight; rest for 15–30 seconds

SET 2: 10 repetitions with middle weight; rest for 15–30 seconds

SET 3: 8 repetitions with heaviest weight; rest for 15–30 seconds

REMINDER

See pages 55–57 for tips on heaviness of weights.

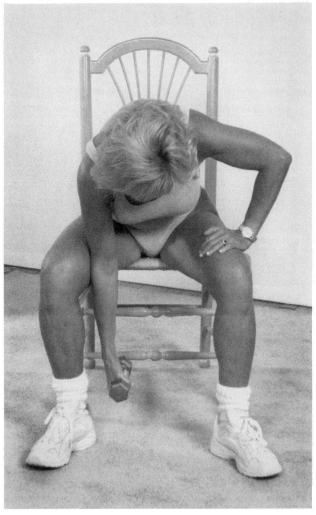

CONCENTRATION CURL: START

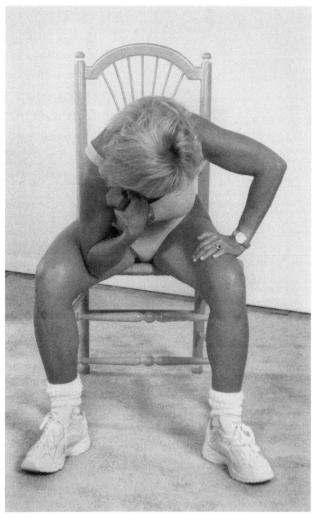

CONCENTRATION CURL: FINISH

Exercise #5: Triceps Kickback

This exercise strengthens, develops, shapes, and defines the entire triceps muscle, and strengthens the underlying bone (humerus). There is a side benefit to the elbow, shoulder joint, and wrist.

STANCE

Stand with your feet a natural width apart. Hold a dumbbell in your working hand, palm facing your body, and bending at the waist and knees. Bend your arm at the elbows so that your forearm is parallel to the floor. You may keep your nonworking hand on your nonworking knee or lean on a bench for balance.

ACTION

Keeping your upper arm close to your body and flexing your triceps as you go, extend your working arm back as far as you can go. Give your triceps an extra flex and return to the start position, feeling the stretch in your triceps muscle. Repeat the movement for the other arm. Do your second and third sets.

TIPS

Don't let your upper arm wander away from your body during the movement. Don't use jerky movements. Maintain a fluid action. Try to keep your upper arm from moving as you work. Only the forearm should be moving.

MACHINES, ETC.

You may perform this exercise using an appropriate pulley device.

SETS, REPETITIONS, WEIGHTS

SET 1: 12 repetitions with lightest weight; rest for 15–30 seconds

SET 2: 10 repetitions with middle weight; rest for 15–30 seconds

SET 3: 8 repetitions with heaviest weight; rest for 15–30 seconds

REMINDER

See pages 55–57 for tips on heaviness of weights and raising weights.

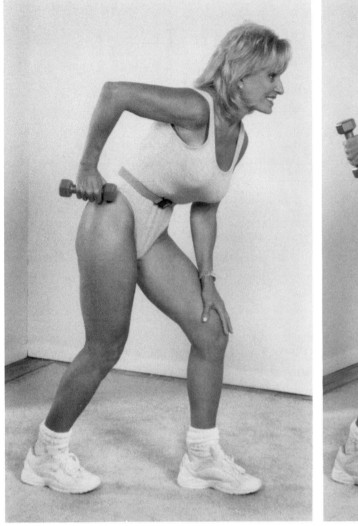

TRICEPS KICKBACK: START

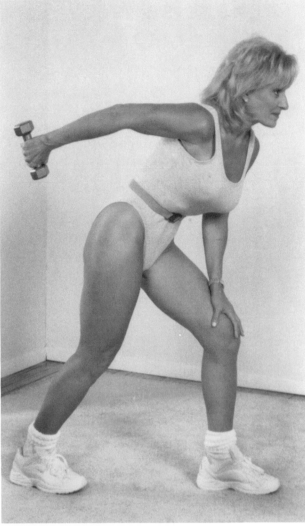

TRICEPS KICKBACK: FINISH

Exercise #6:
Seated One-Arm Overhead Triceps Extension

This exercise strengthens, develops, shapes, and defines the entire triceps muscle and strengthens the underlying bone (humerus). There's a side benefit to the elbow and wrist.

POSITION

Sitting on a flat exercise bench or a chair, hold a dumbbell in your right hand, palm facing the side of your body and your arm extended fully upward. Let your biceps muscle nearly touch your ear. Place your left hand on your right elbow. This serves to support your arm.

ACTION

In full control and feeling the stretch in your triceps muscle as you go, lower the dumbbell behind your head by unbending your elbow and allowing the dumbbell to descend until you cannot go any farther. Keep your upper arm close to your ear and your elbow pointed forward. Without resting and flexing your triceps muscle as you go, return to the start position. Give your triceps muscle an extra flex and repeat the movement until you have completed your set. Repeat the exercise for the other arm. Do your second and third sets.

TIPS

Keep your back straight. Don't hunch over and don't rock. If your elbow is strong enough, you can place your nonworking hand on your triceps instead of on your elbow—to feel it working.

MACHINES, ETC.

You may perform this exercise using any triceps extension machine.

SETS, REPETITIONS, WEIGHTS

SET 1: 12 repetitions with lightest weight; rest for 15–30 seconds

SET 2: 10 repetitions with middle weight; rest for 15–30 seconds

SET 3: 8 repetitions with heaviest weight; rest for 15–30 seconds

REMINDER

See pages 55–57 for tips on heaviness of weights and raising weights.

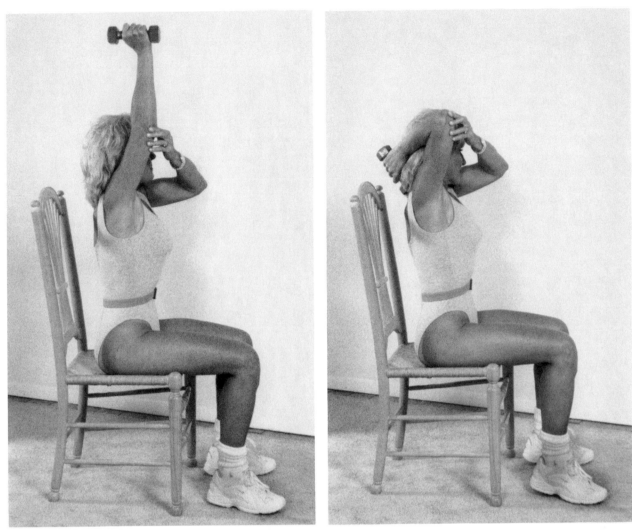

SEATED ONE-ARM OVERHEAD TRICEPS EXTENSION: START   **SEATED ONE-ARM OVERHEAD TRICEPS EXTENSION: FINISH**

Review of Exercises in This Chapter

Arms: Wrist, Biceps, Triceps Workout

WARM-UPS: doggie paw wrist-forearm stretch, scratch-your-back biceps-triceps pull

WRIST EXERCISES

1. Palms-up wrist curl
2. Palms-down wrist raise

BICEPS EXERCISES

3. Standing simultaneous curl
4. Concentration curl

TRICEPS EXERCISES

5. Triceps kickback
6. Seated one-arm overhead triceps extension

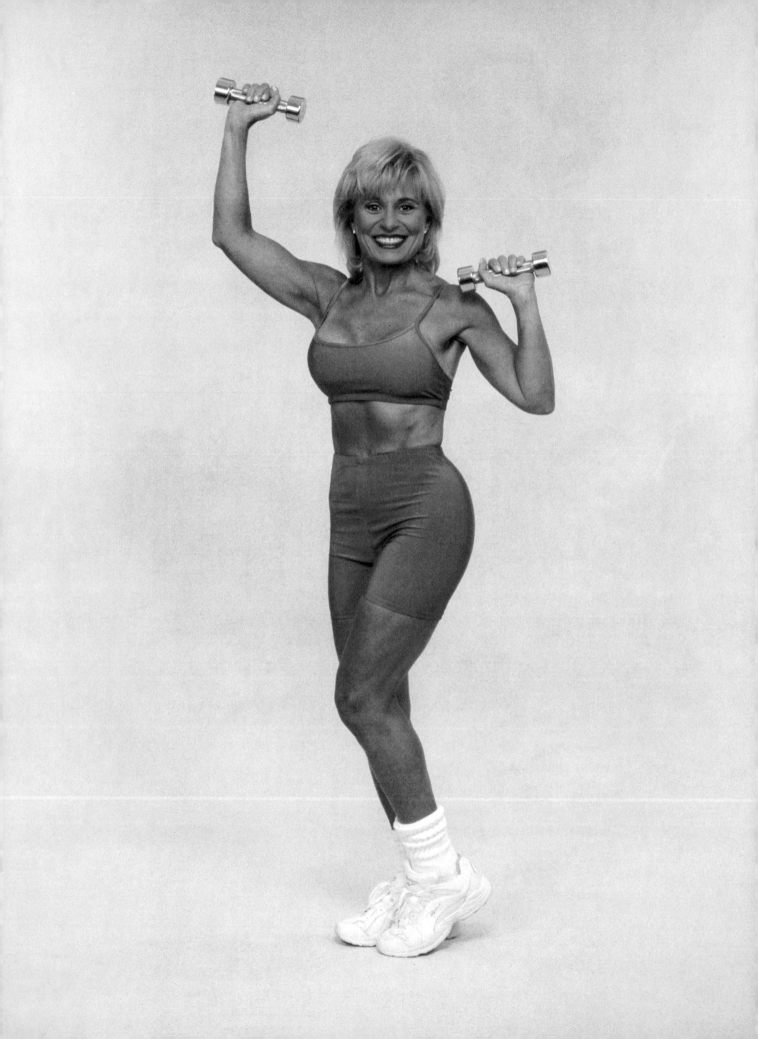

8. Shoulders and Chest for Muscle Tone, Beauty, Bone, and Strength

The last group of exercises for shoulders and chest is by no means "least." Although these two areas do not usually fracture or become targets for improved muscle tone and beauty, they are extremely important.

Beautiful shoulders make all the difference when it comes to a woman's appearance. Well-shaped, defined shoulders give a woman a young, athletic look. In addition, pretty shoulders bring the eye "up" and away from faulty body parts, such as big hips, butt, or thighs.

Many women ask me if they can increase their breast size by working out with weights. The answer is "yes and no." You can change the appearance of your breasts by making them look higher and larger by developing the muscle under your breasts (the pectoral muscles lie just beneath the fatty tissue of the breasts), but that muscle is small and will not significantly increase your breast size. Developing the muscle will make your breasts firmer, however, and in addition you will develop more definition, which will give you greater cleavage and give your breasts a larger appearance.

Of all the bones involved in this workout, the shoulder joints are the most vulnerable to injury and will benefit a great deal from the workout. This is not because the shoulder bones and joints will be strengthened (although they will be) but because the supporting muscles will be strengthened and will protect them from injury. In short, when you have strong muscles, your underlying bones are protected in two ways: You can perform daily tasks and engage in sports, and so forth, with the strength needed to protect your bones from injury, and if you should happen to stumble or fall, your muscles will cushion and protect your bones from fracture. One of the most important aspects of this workout is the development of a strong bone-protecting muscle base.

The shoulder muscle targeted here is the **deltoid** muscle, which originates in the upper area of the shoulder blade and collarbone, and is attached on the bone of the upper arm. The shoulder bones targeted are the **scapula** and **clavicle** (**pectoral girdle**). The scapula has a socket at the end that holds the upper humerus (upper arm bone) and is a vulnerable area to dislocation. The clavicle braces the scapula against the top of the rib cage. Muscles attach to both the scapula and the clavicle.

The **pectoral** muscles of the chest concern us here. These muscles lie under the breasts, originating at the collarbone and running along the breastbone to the cartilage connecting the upper ribs to the breastbone. The chest bones that concern us are the **thoracic cage,** which is composed of the **sternum,** or "breast-bone," and **ribs**. As mentioned in chapter 3, these bones form a protective cage for your heart, lungs, and internal organs. Part of the sternum is attached to most of the ribs. Of the twelve ribs, only the first seven are attached to the breastbone.

As you do your shoulder and chest exercises, be sure to envision the muscles and bones of these areas developing and strengthening. As you follow the exercise instructions and do the workout, remember that you can greatly increase your progress by adding the mind element to the workout (some say by 50 percent). Why not? It doesn't cost you any more time. You're there anyway!

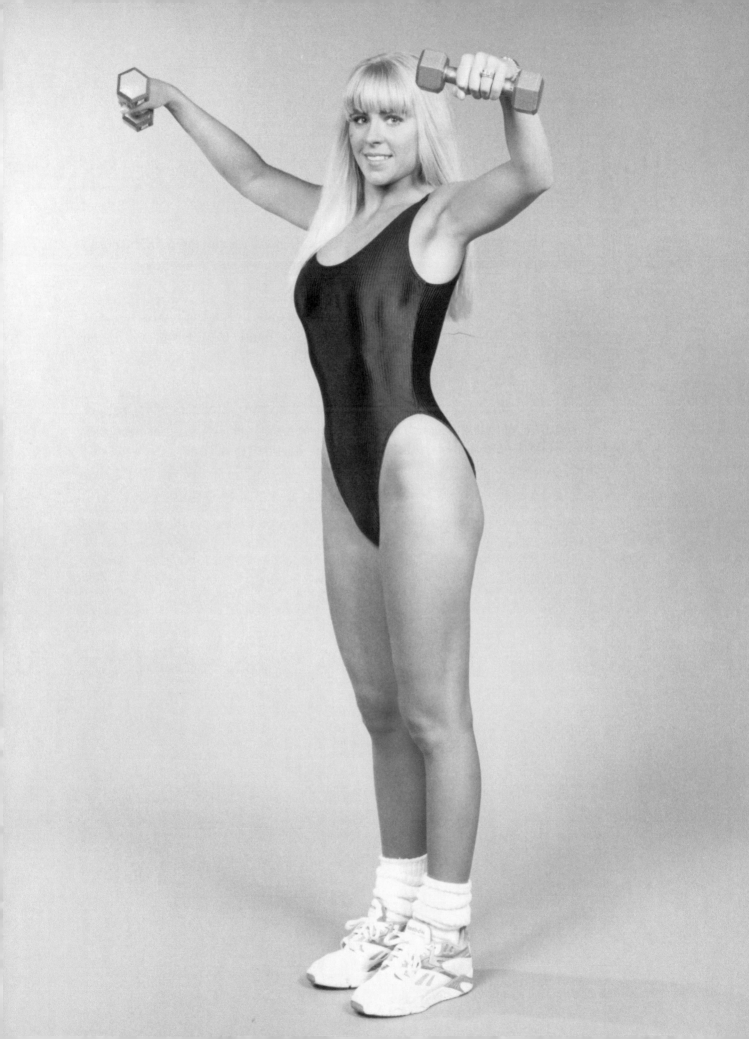

Warm-Up #1:
Hug-Your-Head Shoulder-Back Stretch

This exercise stretch relaxes and strengthens the muscles and bones in the entire shoulder area. There is a side benefit to the upper back and upper arms.

POSITION

Sit on a chair or at the edge of an exercise bench with your feet flat on the floor and your back straight. Place the palms of your hands behind your head, and thrust your elbows forward.

ACTION

Extend your elbows outward and feel the stretch in your shoulders. Make believe you are trying to hold a pencil in the middle of your back on the outermost position. Hold for ten seconds, then return to the start position. Optional: repeat two more times.

TIPS

Don't jerk your arms back. Move in a fluid manner. Don't hold your breath. Breathe naturally.

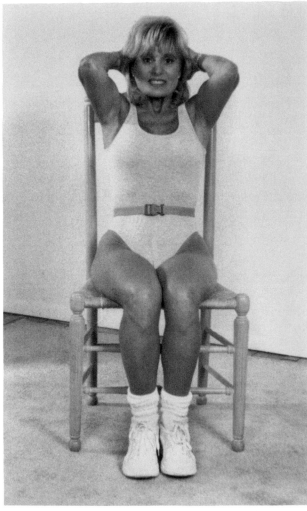 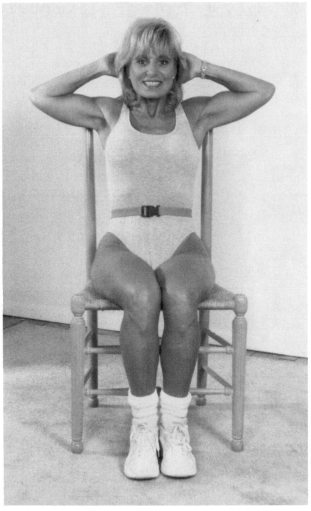

HUG-YOUR-HEAD SHOULDER-BACK STRETCH: START **HUG-YOUR-HEAD SHOULDER-BACK STRETCH: FINISH**

Warm-Up #2: Overhead Towel Chest Stretch

This exercise stretch relaxes and strengthens the muscles and bones of the chest area (pectorals and thoracic cage). There is a side benefit to the shoulders, upper and lower arms, and wrists.

STANCE

Stand with your feet a natural width apart. Hold a towel at either end above your head, with your palms facing forward. (The towel should be large enough so you can move it down behind your back, and you should be holding the towel in a wide enough grip so that you don't strain when moving.)

ACTION

Keeping your arms straight, move your arms over your head and behind you until they are behind your chest at approximately shoulder level. You should feel a full stretch in your chest area. Hold for ten seconds. Optional: repeat two more times.

TIPS

If you don't feel enough of a stretch, you are holding the towel too loosely. Move your hands a little closer together. If you want to use this stretch to relax your shoulders and arms, after pausing at shoulder level, extend your arms all the way down your back until they cannot go any farther.

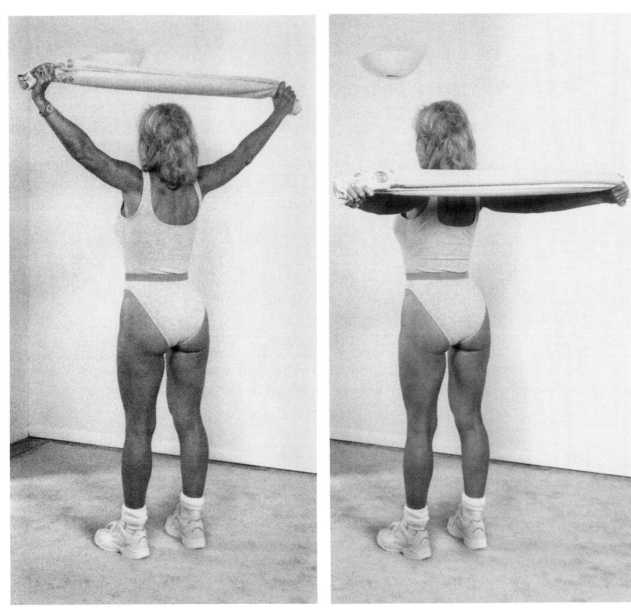

OVERHEAD TOWEL CHEST STRETCH: START

OVERHEAD TOWEL CHEST STRETCH: FINISH

Exercise #1:
Seated Simultaneous Dumbbell Press

This exercise strengthens, develops, shapes, and defines the entire shoulder (deltoid) muscle and helps strengthen the shoulder blade (scapula) and the collarbone (clavicle). There is a side benefit to the trapezius and triceps muscles, and the wrists.

POSITION

With a dumbbell held in each hand at shoulder height, palms facing away from your body, sit on a flat exercise bench or, better, a chair, with your back supported by the back of the chair.

ACTION

Flexing your shoulder muscles as you go, lift your arms upward until your arms are fully extended. Without resting and in full control, return to the start position and repeat the movement until you have completed your set. Do your second and third sets.

TIPS

Maintain full control as you raise and lower the dumbbells—especially when you lower. Don't lock your elbows on the up movement. Do complete movements—all the way up and all the way down. Beware of the temptation to rock back and forth. Keep your body steady. Let your shoulders, not your back, do the work. You may do this exercise standing.

MACHINES, ETC.

You do this exercise on any shoulder press machine.

SETS, REPETITIONS, WEIGHTS

SET 1: 12 repetitions with lightest weight; rest for 15–30 seconds
SET 2: 10 repetitions with middle weight; rest for 15–30 seconds
SET 3: 8 repetitions with heaviest weight; rest for 15–30 seconds

REMINDER

See pages 55–57 for tips on heaviness of weights and raising weights.

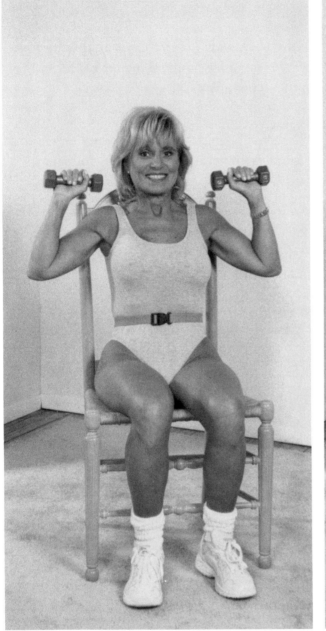

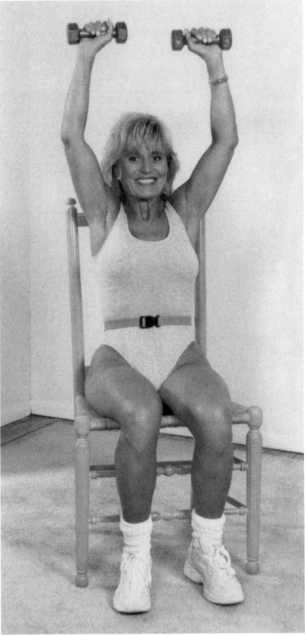

SEATED SIMULTANEOUS DUMBBELL PRESS: START

SEATED SIMULTANEOUS DUMBBELL PRESS: FINISH

Exercise #2: Easy-Does-It Side Lateral

This exercise strengthens, develops, shapes, and defines the entire shoulder (deltoid) muscle and helps strengthen the shoulder joints, shoulder blade, and collarbone. There is a side benefit to the upper arms and wrists.

STANCE

Holding a dumbbell in each hand, palms facing each other and elbows bent at approximately a 90-degree angle, stand with your legs shoulder-width apart.

ACTION

Flexing your shoulder muscles as you go, extend your elbows outward until your upper arms are parallel to the floor. (Your palms will be facing the floor.) In full control, return to the start position and repeat the movement until you have completed the set. Do your second and third sets.

TIPS

After a few weeks you may feel strong enough to advance to the regular side lateral raise. If so, you can eliminate this exercise and replace it with that one or do that one in addition to this one. Don't tense your neck as you work. Don't hold your breath. Breathe naturally.

MACHINES, ETC.

You may do this exercise on any side lateral machine.

SETS, REPETITIONS, WEIGHTS

SET 1: 12 repetitions with lightest weight; rest for 15–30 seconds
SET 2: 10 repetitions with middle weight; rest for 15–30 seconds
SET 3: 8 repetitions with heaviest weight; rest for 15–30 seconds

REMINDER

See pages 55–57 for tips on heaviness of weights and raising weights.

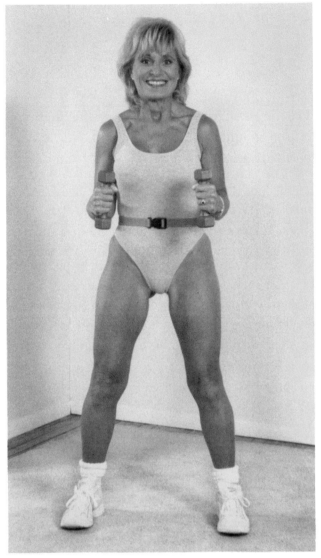

EASY-DOES-IT SIDE LATERAL: START

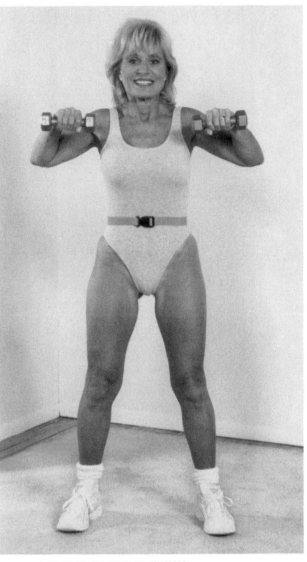

EASY-DOES-IT SIDE LATERAL: FINISH

Variation of Exercise #2: Regular Side Lateral

This exercise strengthens, develops, shapes, and defines the entire shoulder (deltoid) muscle and helps strengthen the shoulder joints, shoulder blade, and collarbone. There is a side benefit to the upper arms and wrists.

STANCE

Stand with your feet a natural width apart. Hold a dumbbell in each hand with your arms extended down and your palms facing each other. The dumbbells should be touching each other at the center of your body.

ACTION

Flexing your shoulder muscles as you go and keeping your elbows slightly bent throughout the movement, make believe you're pouring a pitcher of water. Extend your arms upward and outward until the dumbbells are shoulder height. In full control, return to the start position and repeat the movement until you have completed the set. Do your second and third sets.

TIPS

Beware of the temptation to rock back and forth as you work. Anchor yourself. Don't swing the dumbbells. Let your shoulders, not your back, do the work. If this exercise is too difficult for you, do the Easy-Does-It Side Lateral Raise until that becomes too easy. Try not to go higher than shoulder height.

MACHINES, ETC.

You may do this exercise on any side lateral machine.

SETS, REPETITIONS, WEIGHTS

SET 1: 12 repetitions with lightest weight; rest for 15–30 seconds
SET 2: 10 repetitions with middle weight; rest for 15–30 seconds
SET 3: 8 repetitions with heaviest weight; rest for 15–30 seconds

REMINDER

See pages 55–57 for tips on heaviness of weights and raising weights.

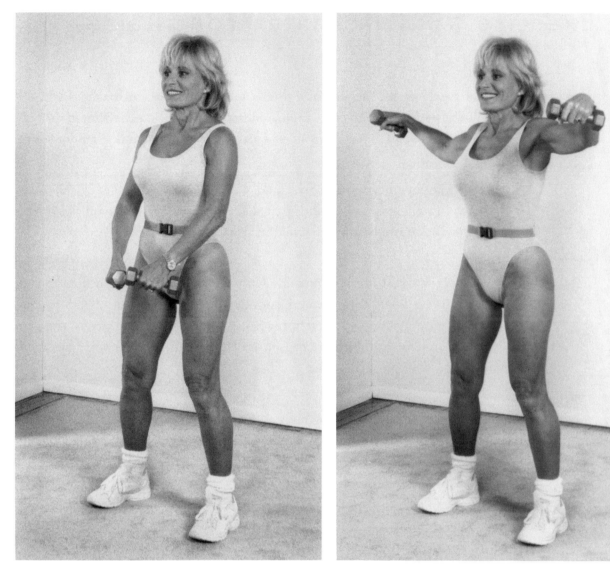

REGULAR SIDE LATERAL: START

REGULAR SIDE LATERAL: FINISH

Exercise #3: Alternate Front Raise

This exercise develops, shapes, strengthens, and defines the entire shoulder (deltoid) muscle, especially the front area, and helps strengthen the shoulder bones (scapula and clavicle). There is a side benefit to the wrists and shoulder joints.

STANCE

With your knees bent very slightly, stand with your feet shoulder-width apart. Holding a dumbbell in each hand, palms facing your body, extend your arms straight down. A dumbbell will be held in front of each thigh.

ACTION

With your elbows as straight as possible without locking them, and flexing your shoulder muscles as you go, extend one arm up until the dumbbell reaches shoulder height. Feeling the stretch in your shoulder muscle, return to the start position. Repeat for the other arm. Continue alternating until you have completed the set. Do your second and third sets.

TIPS

Keep your arms in front of your body throughout the movement. Don't swing the dumbbells to give yourself momentum. Don't rock. Keep your body steady. Lift only to shoulder height. Don't hold your breath. Breathe naturally.

MACHINES, ETC.

You may use a barbell instead of dumbbells and perform this exercise two arms at a time.

SETS, REPETITIONS, WEIGHTS

SET 1: 12 repetitions with lightest weight; rest for 15–30 seconds

SET 2: 10 repetitions with middle weight; rest for 15–30 seconds

SET 3: 8 repetitions with heaviest weight; rest for 15–30 seconds

REMINDER

See pages 55–57 for tips on heaviness of weights and raising weights.

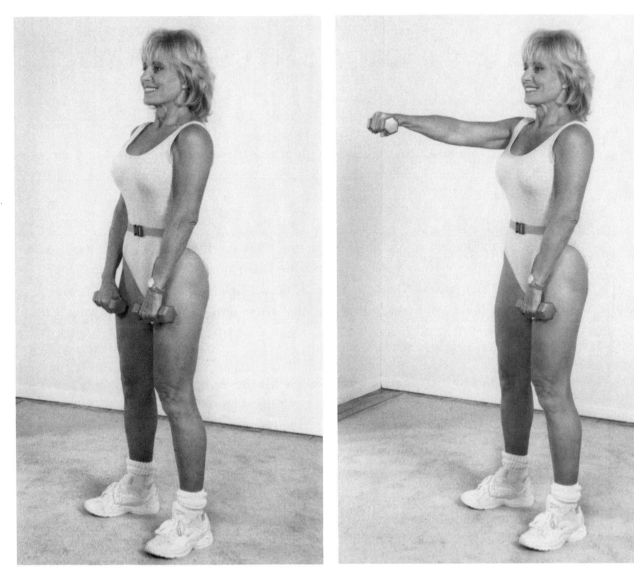

ALTERNATE FRONT RAISE: START

ALTERNATE FRONT RAISE: FINISH

Exercise #1: Dumbbell Bench Press

This exercise develops, shapes, strengthens, and defines the entire chest-breast (pectoral) area and helps strengthen the breastbone (sternum) and rib cage. There is a side benefit to the upper arms, forearms, wrists, shoulders, and shoulder joints.

POSITION

Lie on a flat exercise bench or "step" with a dumbbell in each hand, palms facing away from your body and the inner edge of each dumbbell touching the outer edges of your upper chest-shoulder area. Bend your knees and place the soles of your feet so that you don't arch your back. Press your back into the bench.

ACTION

Flexing your chest muscles as you go, lift the dumbbells above your chest, until your arms are fully extended, but don't lock your elbows. Without resting, return to the start position and feel the stretch in your chest muscles. Repeat the movement until you have completed the set. Do your second and third sets.

TIPS

The dumbbells should be in line with your upper chest in the fully extended position. Remember to fully extend your elbows downward in the down position. Don't cheat yourself by doing half movements. Don't hold your breath. Breathe naturally.

MACHINES, ETC.

You may use the lying bench press machine to do this exercise.

SETS, REPETITIONS, WEIGHTS

SET 1: 12 repetitions with lightest weight; rest for 15–30 seconds

SET 2: 10 repetitions with middle weight; rest for 15–30 seconds

SET 3: 8 repetitions with heaviest weight; rest for 15–30 seconds

REMINDER

See pages 55–57 for tips on heaviness of weights and raising weights.

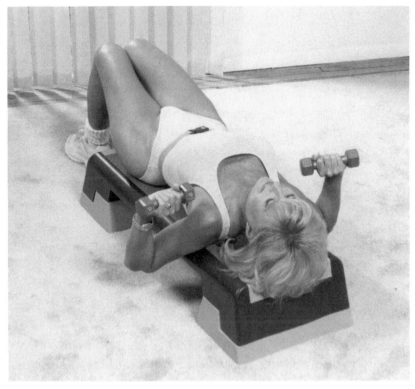

DUMBBELL BENCH PRESS: START

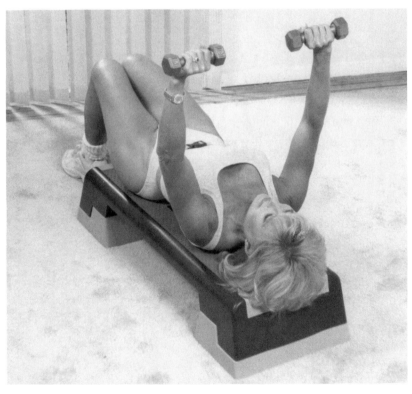

DUMBBELL BENCH PRESS: FINISH

Exercise #2: Easy-Does-It Push-Up

This exercise develops, shapes, strengthens, and defines the entire chest-breast (pectoral) area and helps strengthen the breastbone (sternum) and rib cage. There is a side benefit to the upper arms, forearms, wrists, shoulders, and shoulder joints.

POSITION

Lie in a prone position with your arms shoulder-width apart, the palms of your hands flat on the floor, and your fingers facing forward. Bend your elbows so they are pointed up rather than back. Your feet should be a few inches apart and your toes pointed away from you.

ACTION

Flexing your chest muscles as you go and keeping your knees grounded throughout the movement, extend your arms until your elbows are nearly but not quite locked. Consciously do the work mainly with your chest muscles. Your shoulders will be directly above your hands on the finish position. Return to the start position and repeat the movement until you have completed the set. Do your second and third sets. (Note: This exercise does not use weights because your body is the "weight.")

TIPS

Keep your thighs, buttocks, back, and head in a straight line as you work. Only your knees should be bent, not your back or neck. Continually remind your chest, not your arm muscles, to do most of the work. After a few weeks you may feel strong enough to advance to the regular push-up. If so, you can eliminate this exercise and replace it with that one, or do that one in addition to this one.

MACHINES, ETC.

You may use the seated bench press machine in place of this exercise.

SETS, REPETITIONS, NO WEIGHTS

SET 1: 10 repetitions with no weight; rest for 15–30 seconds

SET 2: 10 repetitions with no weight; rest for 15–30 seconds

SET 3: 10 repetitions with no weight; rest for 15–30 seconds

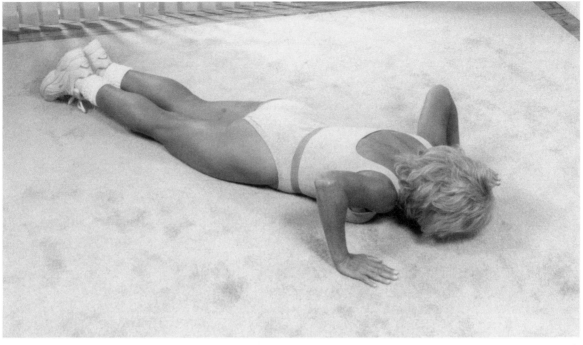

EASY-DOES-IT PUSH-UP: START

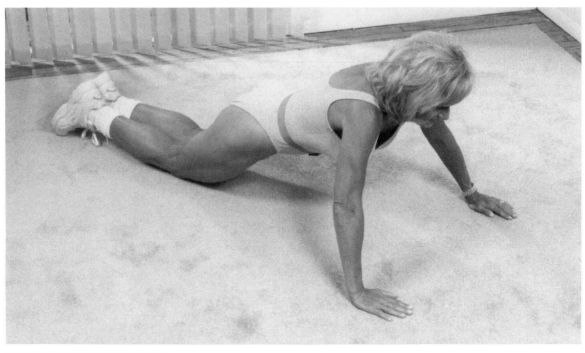

EASY-DOES-IT PUSH-UP: FINISH

Exercise #2a: Regular Push-Up

This exercise develops, shapes, strengthens, and defines the entire chest-breast (pectoral) area and helps strengthen the breastbone (sternum) and rib cage. There is a side benefit to the upper arms, forearms, wrists, shoulders, and shoulder joints.

POSITION

Lie flat on the floor with your arms out, bent at the elbows, and the palms of your hands flat on the floor, fingers facing forward. Your feet should be a few inches apart, with your toes pointed toward the floor.

ACTION

Keeping your entire body straight, letting your knees rise off the floor as you move, and flexing your chest muscles as you go, "tell" your chest muscles to do the work and extend your arms until your elbows are nearly locked and your body is completely off the floor. (The only two body parts that will be touching the floor in the finish position are your toes and the palms of your hands.) In full control, return to the start position and feel the stretch in your chest muscles. Repeat the movement until you have completed the set. Do your second and third sets.

Note: There are no weights to "pyramid," so you will do three sets of ten repetitions.

TIPS

Don't allow your body to take a "swayback" position. Keep your head, neck, back, hip/buttocks, and legs in a straight line as you move. "Tell" your chest muscles to do the work. (Your arms will also be working, but make your chest work, too!) Don't worry if you can only do three or four regular push-ups in the beginning. You will build up over time.

MACHINES, ETC.

This is a very comprehensive and strenuous exercise. There is no real machine equivalent, but the seated bench press comes the closest.

SETS, REPETITIONS, NO WEIGHTS

SET 1: 10 repetitions with no weight; rest for 15–30 seconds
SET 2: 10 repetitions with no weight; rest for 15–30 seconds
SET 3: 10 repetitions with no weight; rest for 15–30 seconds

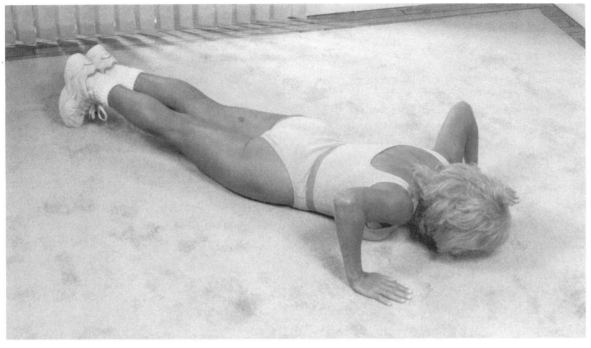

REGULAR PUSH-UP: START

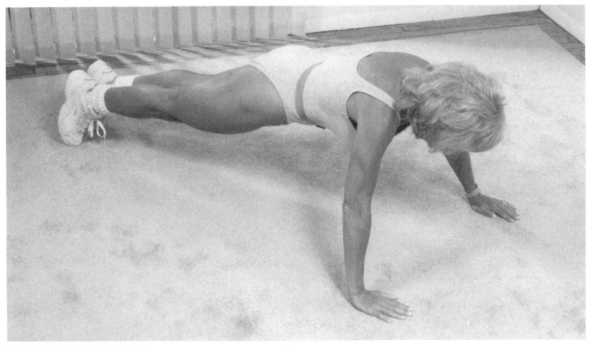

REGULAR PUSH-UP: FINISH

Exercise #3: Dumbbell Fly

This exercise develops, shapes, strengthens, and defines the entire chest-breast (pectoral) area and helps strengthen the breastbone (sternum) and rib cage. There is a side benefit to the upper arms, shoulders, and shoulder joints.

POSITION

Holding a dumbbell in each hand, palms facing each other, lie on a flat exercise bench or "step." Bend your knees and place the soles of your feet flat to prevent your back from arching. Extend your arms straight up, with elbows bent very slightly. The dumbbells should be above the center of your chest.

ACTION

Extend your arms outward and downward in an arclike movement until you feel a complete stretch in your chest muscles. Flexing your pectoral muscles as you go, return to the start position and repeat the movement until you have completed the set. Do your second and third sets.

TIPS

Beware of the temptation to swing the dumbbells out and jerk them back in. Maintain control at all times. Don't lock your elbows. Keep them slightly bent throughout the movement as if they were slightly curved steel bars. Don't hold your breath. Breathe naturally.

MACHINES, ETC.

You may use the pec-dec machine in place of this exercise.

SETS, REPETITIONS, WEIGHTS

SET 1: 12 repetitions with lightest weight; rest for 15–30 seconds

SET 2: 10 repetitions with middle weight; rest for 15–30 seconds

SET 3: 8 repetitions with heaviest weight; rest for 15–30 seconds

REMINDER

See pages 55–57 for tips on heaviness of weights and raising weights.

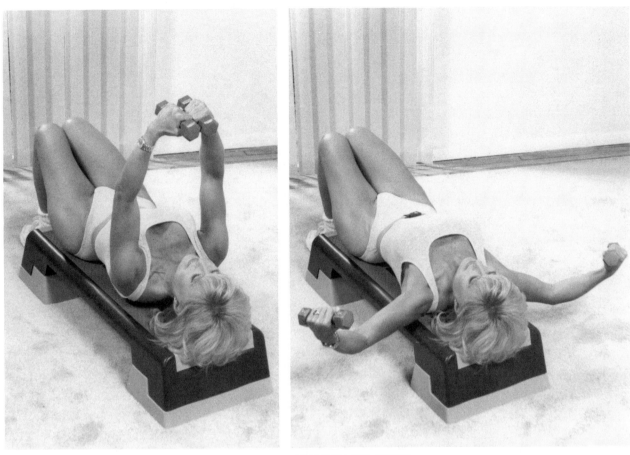

DUMBBELL FLY: START

DUMBBELL FLY: FINISH

Review of Exercises in This Chapter

Shoulder and Chest Workout

WARM-UPS:

hug-your-head shoulder-back stretch, overhead towel chest stretch

SHOULDERS

1. Seated simultaneous dumbbell press

2. Easy-does-it side lateral

2a. Regular side lateral

3. Alternate front raise

CHEST

1. Dumbbell bench press

2. Easy-does-it push-up

2a. Regular push-up

3. Dumbbell fly

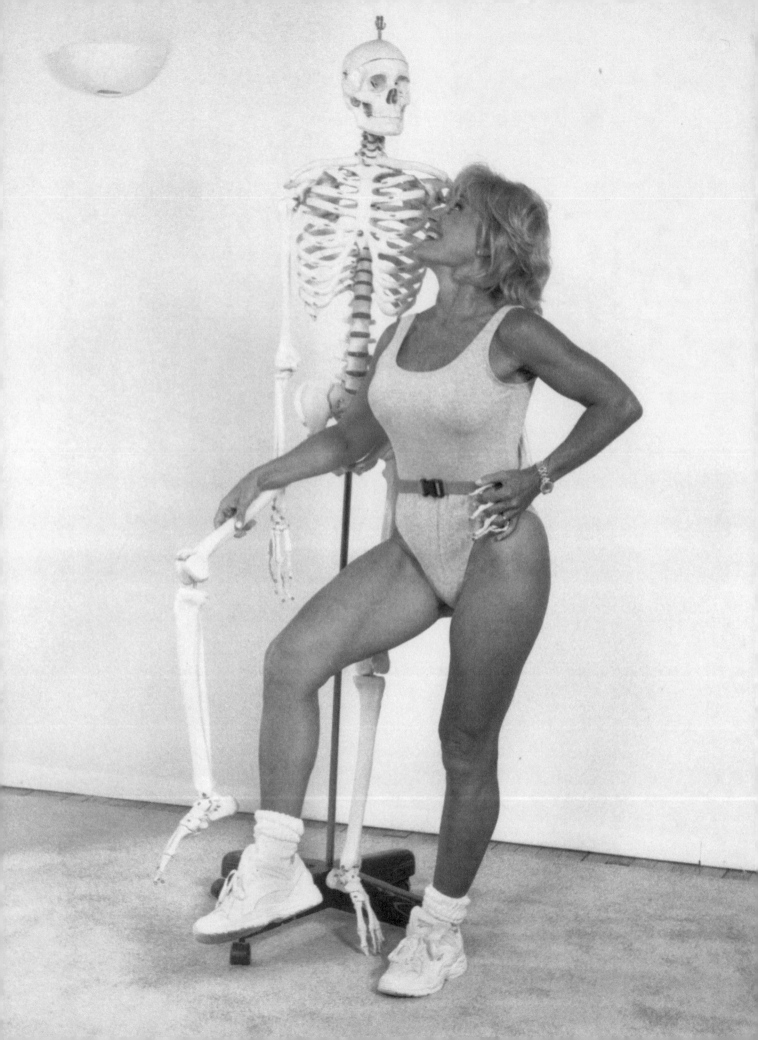

9. Bone-Building Aerobics

Why do aerobics in addition to the weight-training workout? Because the more bone-building activities you perform, the more bone you will build. And since you can get a "triple whammy" from such aerobics (burn fat, improve heart and lungs, and strengthen bone), it's a good idea to pick aerobic activities that put more emphasis on the bone—unless you have a medical problem and the only aerobic activity you can do is swim.

According to The National Osteoporosis Foundation, weight training, climbing stairs, walking, hiking, running, or jogging on the treadmill, downhill skiing, cross-country skiing, low-impact aerobic dancing, and dancing are the best weight-bearing exercises. Stair-step machines, cross-country ski machines, and water aerobics provide somewhat of a weight-bearing aerobic effect.

Some of the above activities are more "aerobic" than others. It is easier to get an aerobic effect from continually climbing up and down a flight of stairs, walking fast, or running or jogging on a treadmill than it is from downhill skiing or dancing. But one can get a full effect from these activities if they are performed in a certain manner. More about this later.

But what about swimming and riding the exercise bicycle and those other seated machines (new ones seem to be coming out every day)? These are not considered *weight-bearing* aerobic activities because they do not "bear the weight of the body." You do burn fat and get an aerobic effect for your heart and lungs, but you do not get the bone-building effect. For the purposes of this book, we are looking for both bone-building and aerobic effects.

Which bones do weight-bearing aerobic activities enhance? These activities challenge the spine, hipbones, and leg bones. The arm and shoulder bones are not really affected by them because your arms and shoulders do not "bear" the weight of your body.

What Is an Aerobic Exercise?

As explained in chapter 3, in order to be considered aerobic, the exercise must utilize the larger muscles of the body, cause the pulse to reach a rate of 60 to 80 percent of its capacity, and stay that way for twelve minutes or longer. The exercise must also be supported by the body's natural flow of oxygen (the word "aerobic" means "with oxygen"). In other words, the exercise must not be so strenuous that you have to take frequent rests in order to catch your breath.

Minimum, Medium, and Maximum Pulse Rates

To figure out your minimum aerobic pulse rate, subtract your age from 220, and multiply the result by 60 percent. For a slightly higher pulse rate, in the medium range, multiply the results by 70 percent. For the maximum challenge, multiply the result by 80 percent. I'll do mine by way of example. I am 54 years old. If I subtract 54 from 220, I get 166. To get my minimum pulse rate, I multiply 166 by 60 percent. The result is 99.6, so I'll say 100. In other words, I must have a pulse rate of 100 in order to be in my lowest aerobic range. If I want to be in my middle range, I multiply my pulse rate by 70 percent: the result is 116.20, or 116. When I multiply by 80 percent for the highest range, I get 132.88, or 133.

Taking Your Pulse the Easy Way

How do you take your pulse? You can find your pulse beat on your wrist or neck, and then count the beats as you look at the second hand of a clock for fifteen seconds. Then multiply the result by four. For example, if I counted twenty-six beats on my wrist in fifteen seconds, I know my pulse is 104—and I'm in my lowest aerobic range.

But is it really necessary to continually monitor your pulse to make sure you're getting an aerobic effect? No. As long as you break into a sweat after about seven minutes, you can be sure that you're in at least the lowest range. In the beginning stages you may want to check your pulse just to get a feel for how hard you have to work to get into your desired range. After that, just enjoy yourself. But if you're the "monitoring" type, monitor away!

"Ease into It" Plan for Any Aerobic Activity

Unless you have already been performing a specific aerobic activity, it's a good idea to follow this "ease into it" plan:

Week 1: three to five minutes

Week 2: five to seven minutes

Week 3: seven to ten minutes

Week 4: ten to fifteen minutes

Week 5: fifteen to twenty minutes

Week 6: twenty to twenty-five minutes

Week 7: twenty-five to thirty-five minutes

Week 8: thirty-five to forty-five minutes

Continue to add five to ten minutes a week until you reach the maximum of one hour. Twenty to forty minutes is plenty of aerobics, however, unless you are in the lowest range and are simply enjoying yourself. Then you can go for an hour. I don't recommend any more than that in one session. I do forty-five to fifty minutes of the stair-stepper or fifty minutes of walking. I used to run, but I'm getting too many aches and pains from it. I hope to resume running twice a week at some point. I find that as I get older, my body is less and less tolerant of all that pounding. But if I don't overdo it and do it every day, my body tolerates it. Recently, I abused running by doing it five days in a row for months at a time. Now I have to lay off for a while. But I've come to love walking!

Why Aerobics Cannot Give You the Ideal Tight, Toned Body of Your Dreams

Years ago many people thought they could get the perfect body shape by just running. Everyone took to the tracks, the streets, the treadmills, the highways and the byways. But what happened? In the end we had a bunch of people with great calves, a healthy heart and lungs, but flabby bodies—and even, in some cases, a "paunch" on the stomach. Other aerobic enthusiasts had other pretty body parts. For example, bikers had well-developed legs and swimmers had pretty backs and shoulders.

The bottom line is that aerobic activities cannot take the place of weight training when it comes to shaping, sculpting, and defining each and every body part. The only body parts that aerobic activities can shape are the particular body parts involved in the activity.

Weight-Bearing Aerobic Activities

Let's talk about specific weight-bearing aerobic activities.

Stair Climbing

I'm talking about actually climbing stairs, not using a stair-stepping device of any kind. You can walk up and down the same flight of stairs in your home—or, better, you can find five to six flights of stairs and continually go up and down. If you're near an athletic field, you can even run up and down the many stairs outdoors—in good or bad weather, depending on your nature. (I used to love to run in the rain, cold, wind, and so forth. Now I wouldn't do it if you paid me!)

Stair climbing is one of the most effective aerobic activities available, not only for heart and lung stimulation but for bone enhancement and calorie burning. If you go two steps at a time, you'll reshape your buttocks muscles. In fact, this kind of stair climbing is the only aerobic activity that has a major effect on the buttocks muscles because you are actually lifting your entire body, using your buttocks muscles, as you climb the stairs two at a time.

Walking

Plain old-fashioned walking. I walk every other morning for about fifty minutes. While I'm walking, I think, meditate, and even pray. I contemplate the sky, the flowers, and the trees—everything in nature. I take the opportunity to thank God for everything I can think of. I could start out in the worst mood, but by the time I get home, I'm always uplifted.

You can schedule your walk early in the morning, or you can do what I often do—put it off until later so it fits into something you have to do anyway. For example, when I have a meeting in New York, rather than take a taxi from one place to another, I'll walk the forty to sixty blocks—and lo and behold, I've walked two to three miles. It takes thirty to forty-five minutes—often the same time as waiting for a cab and sitting in traffic or riding a bus or subway. And by doing it this way, I've saved forty-five minutes of that precious morning time. But I do this only when I'm positive I will have the opportunity to walk later.

It's true that while walking you're unlikely to go past the lower or middle aerobic range, but who cares? You still burn lots of fat, and it's one of the best weight-bearing activities. In addition, walking is easy on your body, and unlike running or jogging, you'll probably be able to do it every day without irritating your joints and hurting your knees, hips, and back.

Hiking

Hiking is really walking but with hiking boots instead of sneakers, and usually over rough terrain rather than on flat ground or a running track. Clearly, you get a better workout from hiking at a brisk pace than if you stroll along and stop to look at rocks, birds, and so on. But even if you do these things, you are still doing a weight-bearing workout. And when you hike, you usually hike for longer periods of time than when you walk or run, so in the long run you burn as many or more calories. And usually it's more fun. It's also more fun to hike with someone than to walk or run with someone because you can talk about what you see on the hike.

Running, Walking, or Jogging on a Treadmill

The advantage of a treadmill is the even surface it provides. You can't fall on a rock or other object, so you're less likely to be injured. Another good thing about a treadmill is *consistency*. You can set the treadmill to a certain speed and slant grade, and then you're forced to keep up the effort. You can't cheat—unless you deliberately change the speed or slant. Outdoors, on the other hand, you can slow down and not even know it. You can also run on flat or hilly ground and have no idea how much of each one you covered.

Another obvious advantage of the treadmill is that you don't have to worry about the weather, safety from attackers, and getting lost. (I'll never forget the time I got hopelessly lost while running in a foreign country!) Also, you can read, watch TV, listen to audiotapes, or watch the fancy treadmill scenery (if you have a really expensive machine).

I like running outdoors in spite of all the advantages of the treadmill. I like to run at my own pace, feel the fresh air, and get in touch with nature.

Running or Jogging Outdoors

Running is faster than jogging! In order to be considered running, you should be doing a mile in no more than nine minutes. Anything slower than that is jogging, but so what? I run about an eight-and-a-half-minute mile.

If you plan to run or jog, the most important thing to do is purchase the best pair of running shoes you can. There are many special shoes on the market, so you have a wide range of choices. But no matter which brand you buy, make sure it is specifically labeled "running" shoe, not "tennis," "walking," or any other type. Running shoes are specifically constructed to absorb the shock of the continual bounce of your body on the ground. If you don't use the proper shoe, you may find yourself with "shinsplints," a painful bone ache that will force you to stop running for months.

One more thing: Try not to run on concrete—at least not for more than a small portion of the run. Instead, run on a running track, dirt, or even asphalt. These materials have some elasticity and are less likely to cause shinsplints or other problems.

Downhill Skiing

Since many exercise specialists now agree that you can get an aerobic effect in even twelve minutes, downhill skiing qualifies as an aerobic activity. While you're skiing, the weight of your entire body is borne by you even though you are using ski poles for balance. In addition, you are burning plenty of calories by sweeping around obstacles, bending around curves, and making stops and starts. Your muscles, shoulders, chest, arms, back, legs, abdomen, and torso are being continually called upon to balance your body and, at the same time, keep it moving over varied terrain.

Cross-Country Skiing

This aerobic activity lends itself to those who want continual action but with less danger. Since it is done on relatively flat terrain, there is little chance of injury. For this reason, it is also more relaxing (if you can relax in cold weather). In fact, cross-country skiing reminds me of hiking—with skis instead of hiking boots.

When you cross-country ski, you bear your own weight and at the same time work nearly every muscle in the body as you negotiate the ground. You don't have to go to a ski resort to cross-country ski. You can do it anywhere there is snow—as long as the ground isn't too hilly!

Low-Impact Aerobics

The great thing about low-impact aerobics is that you can socialize and at the same time burn fat and get your heart and lungs in shape. In addition, because you are moving to the music and the instructor keeps you busy doing one thing and then another, the time goes by so quickly that you don't even realize you were working and sweating for twenty or more minutes. I don't have the time to go to aerobics classes, but whenever I'm vacationing in a spa, I make sure to attend the classes, and I always enjoy myself.

What about high-impact aerobics? They are practically nonexistent today, because of the injuries they cause. Such aerobics involve jumping and landing with full force time and again. I don't recommend them.

Dancing

Whether it's social dancing where you move about to fast music by yourself or ballroom or Latin dance where you move about at a quick pace with a partner, dancing is both weight bearing and aerobic. But as you might imagine, it's effective only for the length of time you are on the move. If you want to use dancing as one of your weight-bearing aerobic activities, I suggest you look at your watch before you start and make up your mind not to sit out a dance until you have danced for as long as your aerobic session is supposed to last—say twenty to thirty minutes.

But what if you stop after, say, ten minutes, rest, and start again? That's not bad at all. We now know that doing aerobic activities in short spurts is almost as good as doing them straight through. And for bone-building purposes they're just as good if not better because you get a second, third, fourth, and fifth wind—and could probably go all night long.

Now to the weight-bearing exercises that have some bone-building capacity but not as much as the above.

Stair-Stepping Machines

Various stair-stepping machines can be purchased for home use. I have one myself. With this machine you can take little steps or deeper steps. The smaller your steps, the less work you are doing and the less "weight-bearing effect" you will get. In any case, you cannot reshape your buttocks with any stair-stepping machine because the machine does not allow you to completely use your own weight.

I like the stair-stepping machine because I can watch TV or a video and work in a relaxed fashion, but I'm not fooling myself. I know that actually climbing the stairs will give me better results. Frankly, though, if I had to do real stairs, I wouldn't do it, so I'm happy that I have a stair-stepper. I do it for forty-five minutes and don't kill myself.

Cross-Country Ski Machines

These machines were quite popular ten years ago and are still quite popular for some. They are considered weight-bearing because the exercise is done in a standing position—arms and legs moving at the same time. People used to believe that they could get their entire bodies in shape by using this machine, but we now know this is not the case.

If you want to use the cross-country ski machine for your weight-bearing aerobic activity, I suggest that you don't use it every day. You would wear down your hard-earned upper body muscles. Instead, use it no more than two or, at the most, three times a week. You can do other aerobic activities on the other days, such as walking, the treadmill, climbing stairs, and so on.

Waterskiing

Believe it or not, waterskiing takes a lot of effort. You must continually balance your body against the water, and to do this, your entire musculature is flexed—tensed against the threat of falling over. Your arms are extended as they hold on to the ropes. Your upper body is continually moving in reaction to the movement of the boat. Your legs bend as you weave in and out of the wake of the boat. You are clearly "bearing" the weight of your body even though you are on the water. If you were swimming, however, you would be borne by the water. That's a different story.

Water Aerobics

Why is water aerobics considered a semi-weight-bearing activity but not swimming? When you swim, you are horizontal the entire time—and the water bears your weight. When you do weight-bearing aerobics, on the other hand, you are vertical—standing up most of the time—and are bearing your weight.

In addition, when you do water aerobics, you exert force by pushing and pulling against the water with your arms, shoulders, and even legs, sometimes while holding a device or wearing one strapped to your arms or legs. This action causes you to work and burn calories while performing a semi-weight-bearing activity.

Non-Weight-Bearing Aerobic Activities

Many other aerobic activities are not weight-bearing, such as riding a bike, horseback riding, rowing a boat, canoeing, or any of the seated devices, including rowing machines. These are perfectly fine for getting a heart-lung aerobic effect and for burning excess fat, but they are not considered bone-building.

Other Aerobic Activities

Other aerobic and semi-aerobic activities that are weight-bearing are not mentioned here, including tennis, golf, volleyball, handball, racquetball, jumping rope, roller-blading, and roller-skating. Use your own judgment.

Obviously golf is not really aerobic, but it is weight-bearing since you are standing a lot. Volleyball, tennis, handball, and racquetball are more aerobic than golf because you are in continual action, but you are interrupted a lot. I wouldn't consider them aerobic, yet they do have some aerobic effect, are good exercise, and, indeed, bear the weight of your body.

Jumping rope, roller-blading, and roller-skating are weight-bearing *and* aerobic but have not yet been officially evaluated by medical experts as to safety and bone-building potential. I imagine that jumping rope has a wonderful bone-building effect, but it may take a toll on the joints due to the pounding. I do it whenever I'm in a hotel room and can't get any other aerobic activity. As for roller-blading and roller-skating, I think they are also weight-bearing, but not as much as walking or running since you are gliding and sliding, and not lifting your weight with each step.

Using the Bone-Building Workout in an Aerobic Way

If you speed-set (don't take rests) or "giant-speed-set" (see page 28 for method), you will get an aerobic effect from working out with the weights using this workout. You should by no means feel obligated to do so, however. In fact, until you get really comfortable with the workout, I don't recommend it. Many people would rather use this workout for sheer weight training and keep their aerobics separate.

Aerobic Exercise Chart: How Many Calories Do You Burn?

AEROBIC ACTIVITY	CALORIES BURNED IN THIRTY MINUTES
Stair Climbing	390
Running	344
Low-Impact Aerobics	300
Jogging	290
Dancing	270
Waterskiing	270
Cross-Country Ski Machines	250
Cross-Country Skiing	230
Downhill Skiing	220
Hiking	180
Stair-Stepping Machines	160
Walking	160

Note: Calorie burning when using stair-stepping machines has been adjusted to the way most people use them—at a gentle pace, taking medium to small steps.

The above table assumes you are putting in moderate effort. If you want to burn even more fat, go faster and flex your muscles—give it that extra push.

Incorporating Your Weight-Bearing Aerobics into Your Weight-Training Plan

If you are going to do aerobics in addition to the bone-building workout, it's a good idea to do these exercises before your workout—as a warm-up. That being said, I must admit that I rarely do. The reason is that quite often I have only a certain amount of time to work out before I have to leave in the morning, and since I know that weight training is the most important, I do it first. Then later in the day, if I have time, I do my aerobics. Other days, when I have time, I do the stair stepper or take a walk, and then do my weight-training workout.

The good news about aerobics is that you can do them any day—three to six days a week or, if you vary them, every day. It doesn't matter if you weight-train on the same day or not. It doesn't matter what type of aerobic activity you do. You can do whichever body parts you are scheduled to do for your weight-training workout; your aerobic activity will not interfere with it.

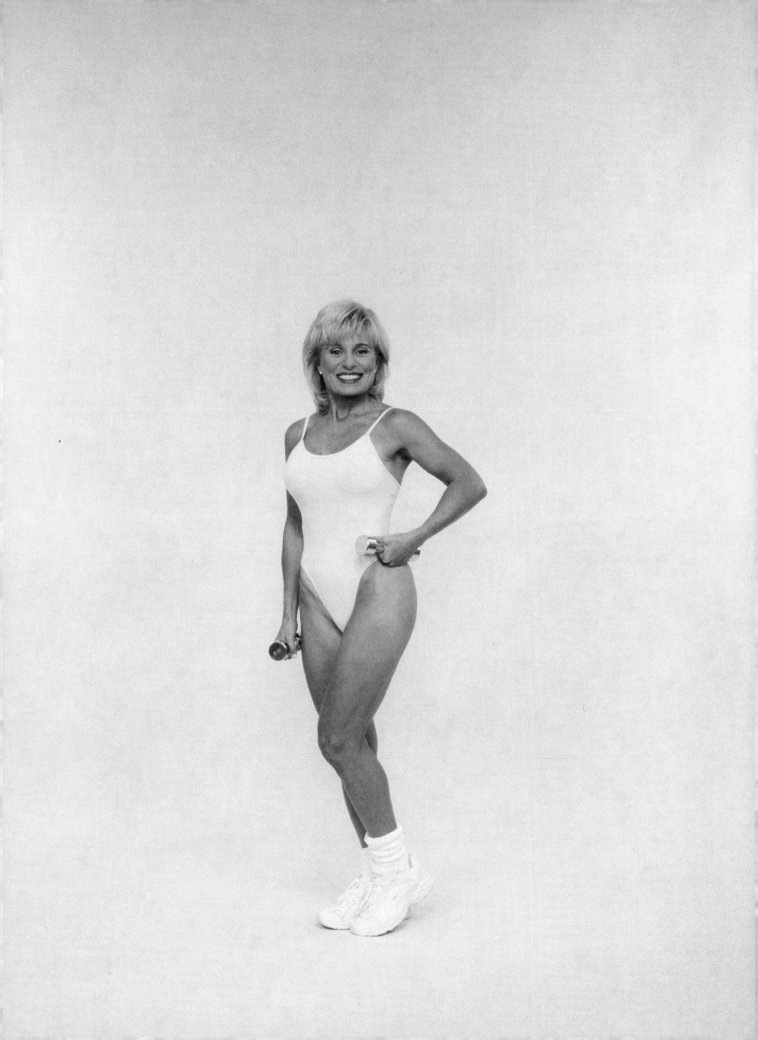

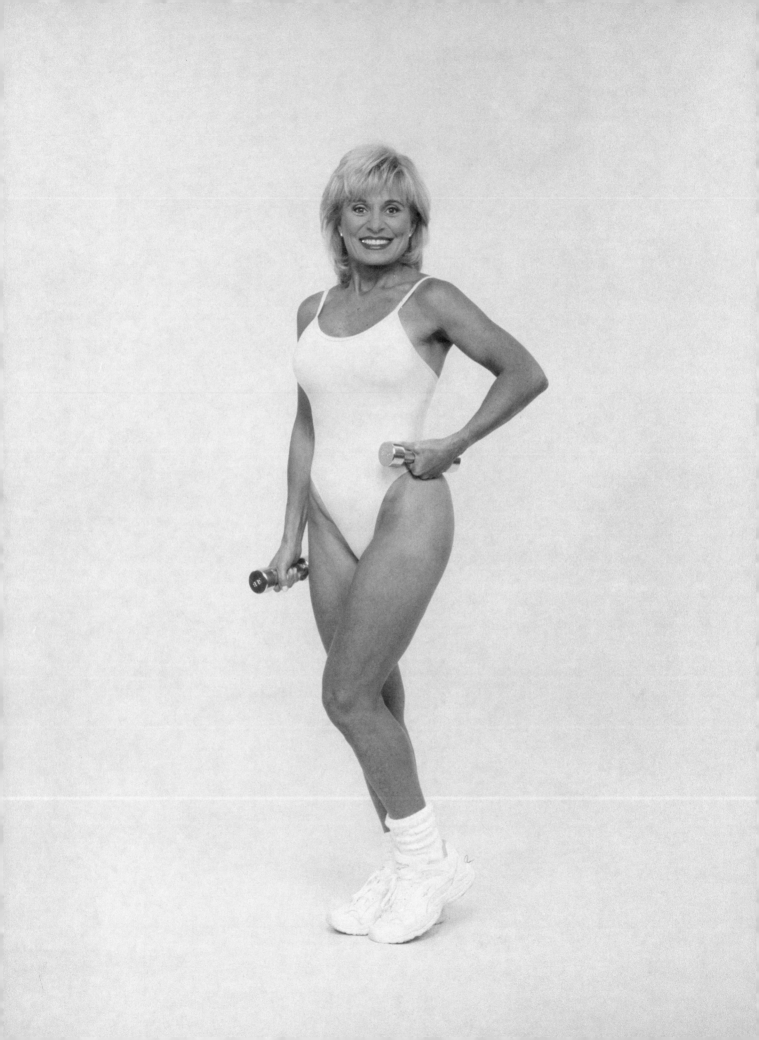

10. Bone-Protecting Keep-the-Fat-Off-the-Body Diet and Nutrition

To be realistic, what good is a bone-protecting nutritional system unless it also keeps excess fat off your body? We are at least as concerned with our appearance as we are with our health, and too much fat also affects our health.

In the following paragraphs you'll learn the basics about good nutrition, with a special emphasis on keeping your calcium intake where it should be. But at the same time you will be given a plan that shows you exactly how to eat the right food combinations for optimum health, energy, and weight loss. If you don't need to lose weight, you'll simply learn how to eat for top strength, energy, and health.

Calcium: What Is It, Why Do We Need It, and How Much Do We Need?

The mineral calcium is stored mainly in the bones (99 percent of it). The other 1 percent is used to do a variety of things to keep us in good health: Calcium helps regulate hormone production, blood clotting, blood pressure, cholesterol (the "good and bad" balance—moving it over to the good), nerve impulses, and heartbeat. Calcium also fights the plaque that causes heart disease and plays a role in mitigating migraine headaches. In addition, calcium helps stir up the fat-burning enzymes that work to control weight gain.

Most of our calcium is stored in the bones. When we are not getting enough calcium for our daily needs, the body will "steal" some from our bones and then, eventually, our bones thin. That's the cause of osteoporosis: Over time, more calcium is removed from the bones than is put in.

Every year about 20 percent of our bone is eroded and replaced by new bone. Old bone is broken down by osteoclasts, and the bone is prepared for remodeling by osteoblasts, which build the bone by filling the spaces in the broken-down bone with new calcium. But if there is not enough calcium to replace the old bone, eventually, bone thins and trouble begins!

Having said that, let's learn once and for all how much calcium you should have in your diet. According to the *National Osteoporosis Foundation*, the total milligrams recommended are as follows:

Children 1 to 10 years	800 to 1,200
Adolescents 11 to 24 years	1,200 to 1,500
Adult women 25 to 49	1,000
Postmenopausal women on estrogen	1,000
Postmenopausal women not on estrogen	1,500
Pregnant or breast-feeding women	1,200 to 1,500
Adult men 25 to 64 years	1,000
Anyone 65 years or older	1,500

Where will you get your calcium? It's always best to try to get it from food. But, frankly, it is nearly impossible to get it all from food every day, so to be on the safe side, you should take a supplement for at least some of it. The leading experts in the field seem to agree that you should try your best with food but take a supplement as an insurance policy. But don't go overboard and take more in supplementation than you should.

The most convenient and commonly used supplement is calcium carbonate. One form of this type of calcium is the popular antacid Tums that can be chewed anytime. Calcium carbonate also comes in capsules and tablets. If you have trouble with this form of calcium (loose bowel movements, constipation, bloating, gas) try taking it right after you eat. Or switch to calcium citrate, which can be purchased in any pharmacy, but don't take it on an empty stomach.

How do you calculate your supplement needs? Think about how much calcium you're getting in your regular diet. Chances are you are getting at least 500 milligrams of calcium. (I certainly hope so.) Say you are a postmenopausal woman not on estrogen. How much should you take? You guessed it: 1,000 milligrams as a supplement. Should you take 1,500 milligrams as a supplement even though you know you are getting 500 in food—just to be on the safe side? No! Don't take excessive calcium. Speak to your doctor to be sure. He or she will guide you in the amount you need. I've provided a meal plan where you get 1,500 milligrams of calcium (see pages 187–88), and you can devise your own meal plans using the information in this chapter.

One more thing: If you need more than 500 milligrams as a supplement, it's a good idea to spread it out during the day. Since most calcium pills come in 500-milligram doses, I suggest you take one in the morning and one at dinner or in the evening. But, I reiterate: Try to get as much of your calcium on a daily basis from foods.

FOOD SOURCES OF CALCIUM	SERVING	CALCIUM (milligrams)	CALORIES	FAT (grams)
Yogurt, plain, no fat	1 cup	452	100	0
Yogurt, plain, low fat	1 cup	415	145	4
Yogurt, fruit-flavored, low fat	1 cup	345	230	4
Milk, skim	1 cup	302	80	1
Milk, 1% fat	1 cup	300	100	3
Ice milk, 3% fat	1 cup	274	225	6
Mozzarella cheese, part skim	1 oz	207	80	4
Ricotta cheese, part skim	4 oz	335	190	9
Cottage cheese, 1% fat	4 oz	69	80	2
Broccoli, cooked from raw	1 cup	136	40	0
Broccoli, cooked from frozen	1 cup	100	50	0
Collard greens, cooked from raw	1 cup	357	65	0
Turnip greens, cooked from raw	1 cup	252	30	0
Kale	1 cup	206	42	0
Spinach	1 cup	168	52	0
Swiss chard	1 cup	128	46	0
Orange juice (calcium-fortified)	1 cup	300	104	0
Soybeans, cooked, drained from raw	1 cup	131	235	11
Tofu, soft	4 oz	108	85	6
Tofu, soft, made with calcium sulfate	4 oz	145	85	6
Sardines, in tomato sauce with bones	3 oz	372	151	10.2
Sardines, in tomato sauce without bones	3 oz	165	151	10.2
Lima beans	½ cup	48	100	0
Kidney beans	½ cup	48	92	0.4

Note: There is some controversy on spinach and turnip greens. They both contain oxalic acid, which can cancel out the benefits of the calcium found in them. It's not a good idea to use them in counting up your calcium for the day, but if you do, cook them with a little vinegar. It may cancel out some of the oxalic acid. Why did I include them here if there is such a problem with them? You might see them listed somewhere, think they are good calcium sources, and use them. For now, don't count on them.

Why did I list the calories and fat grams? You'll need this information when you plan your daily meals (see pages 187–89).

The Calcium–Vitamin D Link

Okay, so you get enough calcium. But unless you get enough vitamin D, your body will not be able to utilize the calcium it ingests. But there's good news: Even if you are exposed to only fifteen minutes of direct sunlight a day (I'm not talking about sunbathing, just having any part of your skin exposed as you walk around), you will get enough vitamin D to utilize your calcium. (And, yes, the vitamin D from the sun comes through even the highest number of sunblock!)

If you don't think you are getting enough sunlight and you don't drink vitamin D–fortified milk, then take a supplement of 400 IU (international units) of vitamin D a day.

Magnesium Is Important, Too!

The mineral magnesium is also necessary to build strong bones—for this reason, most calcium supplements also throw a little magnesium into the mix. Magnesium can be found in fish, whole wheat flour, beans, wheat germ, tofu, pumpkin seeds, and dried apricots.

The Function of Potassium

Although potassium is not a key component in building strong bones, it does work along with calcium to regulate blood pressure. In addition, potassium helps regulate digestive enzymes and carries electrical impulses that keep the heart and other muscles working. You can get potassium from skim milk, wheat germ, dried apricots, raisins, sardines, swordfish, and pumpkin seeds.

Beware of Calcium Drains!

Certain substances can leach calcium from the bones, and it's a good idea to be aware of them. Too much alcohol (more than two drinks a day), too much caffeine (more than three cups of coffee a day), too much salt (more than 2,400 milligrams a day), smoking, too much protein (those high-protein, low-carb diets), too much soda, red meat, or baked goods (all of which have an abundance of phosphoric acid, which depletes calcium), and too much fat (more than 30 percent of total daily caloric intake) drain calcium from your body. Beware and be aware.

How Do You Know if Your Bones Are Thinning? Bone Density Tests

As recently as six years ago, when I went to my doctor and asked for a bone-density test (I was forty-eight), he blew me off, saying, "It's not necessary." Thankfully, in my case, it wasn't because (as I later found out) my bones were quite sturdy. Well, a few years passed, and I kept nagging, and I got the test. (The rest is history; see pages 5 and 6.) Now, thankfully, the medical community is becoming more and more aware of the importance of bone density testing, and most health plans allow for a test at no cost to the patient.

The two most commonly used bone density tests are Dual X-ray Absorptiometry (DXA) and Quantitative Computer Tomography (QCT).

DXA is now the most commonly used bone density test and, in the opinion of many doctors, the most reliable. It uses two beams of light to measure bone density or thickness with little or no risks from radiation. It can measure the bone density of the entire body. QCT also measures bone density or thickness. It's the one I had because it was the only one my doctor had available at the time. It is considered an excellent method of bone measurement but not as good as DXA because it exposes you to a little more radiation than DXA does.

Bone-Enhancing Therapies

Okay. You're getting your calcium from foods and/or supplementing them with tablets, but what about other ways to help your bones? What if you are in menopause and are wrestling with whether to take hormone replacement therapy (estrogen) since it has been proven to slow bone erosion? What about other bone-enhancing therapies such as calcitonin, bisphosphonates, Fosamax, and so on? Let's consider all the options and try to make an informed decision.

Hormone Replacement Therapy

During menopause a woman's estrogen levels decrease. When estrogen decreases, less calcium is absorbed by the bone, and bone density decreases. For this reason many women eventually get osteoporosis. Since this was not my situation—I was already three years into menopause, and my bone density was double the density of women my age because of working out with weights—I was dead set against it.

But for almost a year now, I've been taking HRT (hormone replacement therapy, a combination of estrogen and progesterone), and it's the best thing that ever happened to me. Let me explain why. I didn't mind enduring the hot flashes and night sweats. (Well, I minded, but I figured I would just tough it out.) I didn't mind the irritability and the lack of a sex drive. I didn't even mind the fact that my skin was becoming leathery.

What I did mind was that as time went on, I suffered from such an ennui, a lack of energy, a melancholia, a near depression (although I didn't identify it as such at the time) that it got to the point where it would take an act of will for me to get up out of a chair and type an envelope.

Because of years of self-discipline, I managed to function and even do more than many young energetic women, but it was taking everything I had to do it. Soon I wasn't able to keep it up. I found myself taking shortcuts, turning down business opportunities, being what I called lazy. My outlook for the future became bleak. I began to think of "the end" of it all. I found myself looking into the valley of the shadow of death.

I was melancholy when alone, but in public I somehow managed a near normal appearance of joy, and it wasn't put-on. People cheered me, but whenever possible I would avoid them if I could—for days and even weeks. All the time I was praying, "Help. I'm drowning." I even went to therapy and considered but quickly rejected the idea of antidepressants.

Then one day while skimming some books on estrogen, I noticed that they all agreed there is no short-term risk if you take estrogen. I thought about trying it for a month or two, all the time expecting to drop it. What happened to me was amazing. In a matter of hours I was putting on makeup, wearing high heels, and feeling very energetic. I went shopping at the mall and was quite cheerful. Part of me was looking at myself "outside myself" and thinking, "You're quite happy going shopping. Isn't this out of character?" (I always got depressed when shopping, even before menopause.)

I went through my day blissfully, and at dinner I started to think, "Hey, I haven't felt like this in years." Then it dawned on me that it could be the estrogen. I began to wonder who the shriveled-up, burned-out woman was who had taken over my body. It now seemed as if she had fallen off and was lying on the floor, and I had been transformed into my young, energetic, positive self.

Estrogen for me was a lifesaver. It gave me back my will to live when I didn't even realize I had lost it. But what's more, everyone I see who hasn't seen me since I started taking estrogen (it has now been almost two years) says, "You look ten years younger. What did you do?" My skin is smoother and softer. My hair is shinier and silkier. And what's more, I lost weight! I had actually gained about five pounds from the estrogen, but my will was back, my motivation, my energy. So I perked up and followed my own diet, and I've kept the weight off for over a year.

Why didn't I take estrogen earlier in the game, and why doesn't every woman? For one thing, most doctors don't emphasize the effect of estrogen on mood and energy but instead talk only about its ability to preserve bone and lower the risk of heart disease. My doctor had been nagging me to take estrogen for years, but I had to find out for myself that for me estrogen was the best anti-depressant available.

The real reason I hesitated was the risk. Studies come out every year warning that estrogen may increase the risk of breast and uterine cancer. Let's face it, until the dust settles, there is a shadow of doubt over the safety of taking estrogen. But I'm on the lowest dose, and for me it's worth the risk. You'll have to make your own decision.

Estrogen prevents further erosion of bone density, but it does not in and of itself increase bone density. If you decide to take estrogen, your doctor will also prescribe progesterone with it to protect the uterus. (If you've had your uterus removed, progesterone isn't necessary.) You can take estrogen and progesterone in the form of pills or a skin patch. I take the pills.

Calcitonin

Calcitonin is a hormone produced by the thyroid gland. A synthetic form is used for hormone replacement. The hormone works to prevent bones from further thinning by slowing down the activity of osteoclasts (the cells that break down bone). It is administered either by injection or nasal spray. Some studies show there is a *slight bone density increase* with calcitonin therapy. Calcitonin is also used as a pain reliever for fractures caused by osteoporosis. Bisphosphonate is very similar to calcitonin and works the same way to prevent the osteoclasts from breaking down bone.

Fosamax

Fosamax is the brand name for aldronate, a drug that came on the market in 1995. It is not a hormone but works the same as calcitonin to hinder osteoclasts from doing their work. This drug has been proven *to increase bone density*, whereas estrogen, calcitonin, and bisphosphonates have not been proven to do so (but have been proven to stop further bone erosion).

If these drugs prevent bone erosion and in some cases even increase bone density, why doesn't every woman take them? There are often side effects, such as nausea, moodiness, facial flushing, and so on. Each person responds differently. If you are thinking of taking any of the above, speak with your doctor, read up on it, and make the right decision for you.

The Total Nutritional Picture

Now that you know all about bone-enhancing foods and bone-assisting therapies, what about the rest of your dietary needs? How can you eat plenty of food, enjoy your life, and be not only energetic and healthy but also keep excess fat off your body? First, some basic food facts, then a specific eating plan.

What Are Calories?

Calories are units of chemical energy released to your body when you eat food. The simple equation is to eat just the right amount of calories, and your body will use up the energy released. You will neither gain nor lose weight. Consume too many calories, and your body will store the excess in the form of fat. Keep on consuming too many calories, and you will keep adding to the storehouse and get fatter and fatter. The body's favorite storehouses are the hips, buttocks, thighs, and stomach. Consume fewer calories than you need, and your body uses up the fat stored in those storage bins. But how do you do it? How do you lose the excess pounds?

You already know that you can burn extra calories twenty-four hours a day if you increase your metabolism by working out with weights (as discussed on page 8). You also know that you can burn extra fat by doing the aerobic activities discussed in chapter 9. Now we'll deal with the nutrition part—or, dare I say, "diet."

You can get rid of the storehouse of fat by consuming fewer calories than you burn and, at the same time, eat nutritious, delicious foods that will keep your body healthy, happy, and energetic. There will be no punishment, just some re-learning. The pounds of fat will melt from your body (a pound for every 3,500 calories you remove from the fat storage bank). Easy does it. A pound, a pound and a half, two pounds a week, sometimes less. Your body will not even know it's happening, so it will not fight you. You'll get it off and keep it off—once and for all.

Yes, Calories Do Count, but Fat Calories Are an Issue

You may have heard that as long as you keep your fat intake low, you can eat as much as you want. Well, it's not true. You do have to keep your fat intake low, but at the same time you must be aware of other food issues. Let me explain.

There are 9 calories in each gram of fat, but protein and carbohydrate have only four calories per gram. The picture is clear: Fat is twice as fattening as the other food elements. In addition, fat uses up only 3 percent of its own calories in digestion, while protein and carbohydrate use up about 15 to 20 percent of their calories in digestion. So when you eat fat, you do get fatter than when you eat other food elements. For example, if you eat 100 calories' worth of olive oil, 97 of those calories are put in your energy expenditure account for use, whereas if you eat 100 calories of brown rice, only 80 of those calories are put in your energy expenditure bank for use.

Why We Need Some Fat in the Diet—and How Much We Need

If you cut your daily fat intake so that it is below 10 percent of your total daily caloric intake, you will feel a gnawing hunger all the time and will keep returning to the refrigerator and food cabinets, looking for food. You will keep eating pasta, breads, rice, vegetables, and fruits, and still never be satisfied. Why? You can't fool Mother Nature. In order to be healthy, the body needs a minimum of 10 percent of the total daily caloric intake in fat.

I found this out recently when I wrote my diet book *Eat to Trim.* I always had trouble keeping that last seven pounds off and wouldn't fight the feeling. Off season, I would overeat. I discovered why when I worked with the top nutritionist from the Pritikin Longevity Center. She pointed out that even the Pritikin diet, which is notoriously low in fat, allows dieters to get 10 percent of their calories from fat. She suggested that I check my diet and make sure I was getting—if I was on, say, a 1,500-calorie diet—at least 15 grams of fat a day.

When I analyzed my diet, I realized I was getting only 9 grams of fat a day. I revised my diet, increased the fat to 15 grams, and, wow, what a miracle. I was no longer hungry all the time. I could relax and not hover over the food cabinets and refrigerator thinking about what to eat. And, indeed, I composed my book around that principle.

In fact, I experimented further and found that often I should consume more than the 10 percent minimum—usually 15 percent—or a little higher (15 to 25 grams of fat a day) in order to lose weight without feeling constant hunger. I've provided you with exactly that diet in this chapter.

But why does the body demand that we eat at least a minimum of fat? We need it for our health. We need a certain amount of fat to cushion our internal organs and for our cell membranes and sex hormones. In addition, we need fat in order to make use of calcium and vitamins A, D, E, and K.

Daily Fat Allowance: 15 to 25 Grams

Rather than burden you with counting percentages for fat or any other item in your diet, all you have to think about is adding up fat grams. As long as you keep your daily fat intake to 15 to 25 grams a day, you'll satisfy the percentage. This frees you to pick and choose your fat for the day without obsessing about what percentage of fat a given food has.

Where will you get your allowed fat grams? You will get most of them from protein and dairy; in fact, you'll have to deliberately choose the low-fat dairy products at times, as opposed to the no-fat dairy products, in order to make sure that you get your minimum amount of fat grams. You may on occasion even use half a teaspoon of canola oil to fulfill your daily fat requirement.

I'm not going to give you a list of foods to eat for fat since you will find that in your protein and dairy lists, but I am now going to give you the following:

FORBIDDEN FAT-FOODS LIST

fried foods

lard, butter, margarine, oil (except canola or olive oil in very small quantities to fulfill fat allotment)

croissants, doughnuts

peanut butter, mayonnaise, fat-containing salad dressings (except on rare occasions to fulfill fat allotment)

avocados, olives

potato or corn chips, nuts, seeds

full-fat ice cream, sour cream, cream cheese, cookies, cake

all dairy products over 1 percent fat

pork, beef, veal, bacon

But what about "good fat"? Can't you eat that in abundance and not get fat? No. Even though you may have heard that olive oil and canola oil won't hurt your heart, they will make you as fat as any other fat. Having cleared that up, let's talk about the difference between "good" and "bad" fat.

The fats that are bad for your heart are called *"saturated fats."* These fats become solid or semi-solid at room temperature—just as they will in your arteries, clogging them so that the blood cannot get through to your heart. These are found in animal products such as red meat and egg yolks, full-fat dairy products, and tropical oils such as palm oil and coconut oil, and cocoa butter.

Another group, "trans fats," are the synthetic cousins of saturated fats. They are just as bad because although they are, technically speaking, "unsaturated," they clog the arteries. This group includes partially hydrogenated oil, which is often found in potato and corn chips, crackers, cookies, granola bars, fried foods, and margarine. Yes, margarine is out! (It would be anyway because it is fat, but now you know it clogs the arteries.)

The good fats don't tend to clog your arteries and are categorized into two groups: monounsaturated and polyunsaturated. *Monounsaturated* fats—olive, canola, and peanut oil, avocado, and almonds—do not clog your arteries, and neither do the *polyunsaturated* fats: corn, safflower, sesame, soybean, and sunflower oils, and walnuts.

Before we leave the subject of good fats, I want to talk about *omega-3 fatty acids*, which help prevent blood clotting, atherosclerosis, rheumatoid arthritis, psoriasis, and other inflammatory conditions. I recommend this fat for your diet—but in very small amounts. You can have a few ounces of salmon, sardines, or mackerel every so often to fulfill this need. Tuna also has a small amount of this important nutrient.

What About Cholesterol?

Cholesterol is not a fat but a waxy substance produced in the liver and obtained in the diet. Our brain, liver, blood, nerve linings, and cell membranes are partially formed of cholesterol. In addition, cholesterol helps create vitamin D and bile, as well as our adrenal and sex hormones. How much cholesterol should we have in our diet? No more than about 300 milligrams a day!

The reason we think of cholesterol as a fat is that it can behave like a fat and clog our arteries. It is the cholesterol found in saturated fat that causes the problems. Red meats such as beef, pork, lamb, and veal; organ meats such as kidney, brain, and liver; poultry skin; lunch meats such as salami, sausage, and bacon; full-fat dairy products and egg yolks all contain cholesterol.

Ironically, it is not the foods that have a high cholesterol count—such as shrimp, squid, eel, crayfish, and conch—that do the damage. These foods have a high cholesterol count but a very low fat content; they are low in saturated fat. In other words, it is the saturated fat that is the problem, not the cholesterol count in a given food. You won't have to worry about saturated fat if you follow this diet; you won't have any of it in your diet except in small amounts in the few egg yolks or white meat poultry allowed.

But what about the whole issue of "good" (high-density lipoprotein, or HDL) and "bad" (low-density lipoprotein, or LDL) cholesterol? The bad cholesterol clogs your arteries. Interestingly, the good cholesterol is actually helpful to the arteries; it unclogs them by removing the bad cholesterol. In reality, you should be more concerned with the amounts of each cholesterol in your system than with the total cholesterol count. You can do this by taking a "fractionated" cholesterol test and getting an "index." The lower your index, the better. Here is how it works: Your total cholesterol count is determined, then your good and bad is evaluated separately. Your total cholesterol is divided by your bad cholesterol, and you have your index. By way of example, I'll do mine.

My total cholesterol is 176. My HDL is 54, and my LDL is 122. In order to tell my index, I divide my total cholesterol count, 176, by my good cholesterol, which is 54. The index turns out to be 3.25. An index of 4.0 or lower is considered excellent.

Protein: Two to Three Portions a Day

Remember, I said you will get much of your required fat allotment from your protein. Let's talk about the function of protein in the human body. Protein is so important to our health that it has been called the "building blocks" of the body. Your muscles, internal organs, skin, hair, nails, and blood consist mainly of protein. Protein is used to repair the body. It also affects the production of the hormones that control metabolism, growth, and sexual development, and helps regulate the acid-alkaline balance of the blood and tissues as well as the body's water balance.

Protein consists of twenty-two elements called "amino acids." The human body is capable of producing fourteen of these amino acids and does not need food or any outside source for help, but the remaining eight amino acids must be obtained from specific foods. The foods that have the eight essential amino acids are called "complete protein" foods. Complete protein foods are poultry, fish, milk, milk products, eggs, or a combination of rice and beans, or corn and milk (also red meat, but you won't be eating that now).

Your body needs a minimum of about 60 (some say as low as 45) grams of protein a day if you are a woman. As long as you're eating the low-fat protein, you can consume as much as a gram of protein for a pound of body weight. You can do this because the protein is low in fat and will not make you fat, and because you will not be getting the bulk of it from animal sources. Also, once you start working out with weights, you may find that your body tends to crave a little more protein. We can't prove it needs more yet, but I believe someday we will. Now let's take a look at some sources of protein.

All poultry is without skin and cooked without fat. The fat grams are listed for your convenience.

	GRAMS OF FAT	GRAMS OF PROTEIN
POULTRY (4 OUNCES COOKED)		
Turkey breast	1	34
Turkey drumstick	4.5	33
Turkey thigh	5	31
Chicken breast	4.5	35
Chicken drumstick	6.8	37
Chicken thigh	5	31
FISH (4 OUNCES)		
Mahi-mahi (dolphin fish)	0.8	20.8
Haddock	1	23
Cod	1	26
Abalone	1	16
Sole	1	19
Pike	1	25
Scallops	1	26
Tuna in water	1	34
Squid	1.8	20
Flounder	2.3	34
Red snapper	2.3	26
Sea bass	3.4	25
Halibut	4	31
Trout	4	30
OTHER SOURCES		
Low-fat yogurt (4 ounces)	2	6
No-fat yogurt (4 ounces)	0	7
1% fat milk (8 ounces)	3	8
Skim milk (8 ounces)	1	8
1% cottage cheese (4 ounces)	1	14
No-fat cream cheese (2 tablespoons)	0	2

No-fat cheese (1½ ounces)	0	9
No-fat ice cream (½ cup)	0	2
Egg whites (3)	1	9
*Beans (½ cup)	1	9
*Soft tofu (½ cup)	6	10
*Firm tofu (½ cup)	11	19

* Vegetarian source of protein.

More Protein: Soy Products

Soy products are available in two forms: bean and milk. There are three forms of bean soy: tempeh, miso, and soy flour. Tempeh is made from condensed fermented soybeans. Half a cup has 15.5 grams of protein and 6.4 grams of fat. Miso, a soybean paste made from fermented soybeans and rice (or barley), has 16.3 grams of protein and 8.4 grams of fat per half cup. Soy flour, composed of ground soybeans, is 29.4 grams of protein a cup, and 17.6 grams of fat per half cup, but it can be defatted and have 47 grams of protein a cup and 1.2 grams of fat.

Soy milk has about 80 grams of protein but 4.6 grams of fat. Tofu, curdled compressed soy milk, is a better source of protein. It comes in either soft or hard form. The hard form has had the water removed and is more calorie dense. The soft tofu has 6 grams of fat and 10 grams of protein for half a cup, while the same amount of hard tofu has 11 grams of fat and 19 grams of protein.

Carbohydrates: Simple and Complex

Carbohydrates fall into two divisions: simple and complex. These divisions divide into other branches: simple "refined" and simple unprocessed, limited complex, and unlimited complex.

Carbohydrates supply energy to your body and brain. Simple carbohydrates such as fruit release most of their energy immediately, leaving little for later on when you may need it. Complex carbohydrates, on the other hand, provide gradually released energy that can last for hours.

The simple processed or "refined" carbohydrates are sugars such as those found in white flour, sugar, and the products made from them. Sugar includes any food that contains sucrose, glucose, dextrose, fructose, maltose, sorbitol, or xylitol.

These are not good for you and should be kept to a bare minimum because when taken in excess, they tend to hinder your body's ability to burn fat. When you consume a sugary or white-flour food, glucose is pumped into your bloodstream at a rapid rate. Your insulin level goes sky high, hindering the enzyme responsible for pulling fat from your fat cells (hormonesensitive lipase) from doing its work. The end result is that fat remains in your cells, and your body is forced to burn carbohydrates in its place. For this reason, you are allowed a very small amount of sugary or white flour foods.

Juice can have the same effect as straight sugars when it comes to hindering your body's ability to burn fat, so it's much better to eat the fruit than drink the juice, although a glass of juice is fine on occasion. Watch out for sugar-free foods. They may be loaded with fat—and, in any case, they do have calories.

Now let's talk about complex carbohydrates, the ones that provide gradually released energy for hours. These can be divided into two categories: limited (bread, cereal, pasta, rice, corn, peas, beets, and potatoes) and unlimited (all other vegetables). The limited complex carbohydrates are higher in calories than the unlimited (that's why they are limited). The unlimited, lucky for all of us, are so low in calories and so good for our health that we can eat as much of them as we want, day or night. Since the stomach holds only two pounds of food at a time, we can literally "fill up" on these unlimited carbs and never have an empty stomach if we don't want to.

Speaking of "filling up" on food, a word about caloric density is in order. Caloric density is the number of calories per weight of a given food. Low caloric density foods weigh more but have relatively low calories for their weight. They fill your stomach without causing you to eat too many calories. These foods are found in both limited and unlimited categories. For example, pasta, rice, potatoes, sweet potatoes, yams, and hot cereals are examples of low caloric density foods that you can eat in limited quantities. By way of contrast, cold cereal and whole wheat bread are examples of food with higher caloric density that can be eaten in the limited complex carbohydrate category. For foods that can be eaten in unlimited quantity, brussels sprouts and cauliflower will fill you up (low caloric density) much faster than will escarole or lettuce (higher caloric density). Think of it this way: lower weight equals higher caloric density. "If I want to feel full, I'll eat foods that weigh more—and make my stomach feel full faster."

Now let's talk about how much you can eat of the simple carbohydrates, limited complex carbohydrates, and then unlimited complex carbohydrates.

Simple Carbohydrates: You should have two to four servings of fruit or fruit substitutes a day.

You will get most of your simple carbohydrates from fruit, but occasionally you can have juice, candy, jelly, jam, or low-fat baked goods.

A serving consists of one of the following:

1 medium apple	4 apricots	1 cup berries (any kind)
1 small banana	20 grapes	1 cup papaya
1 medium pear	3 kumquats	1½ cups strawberries
1 large kiwi	3 persimmons	1½ cups watermelon
1 small mango	2 plums	½ cantaloupe
1 large nectarine	2 fresh prunes	½ grapefruit
1 large orange	2 tangerines	¼ large pineapple
l large peach	15 large cherries	½ large plantain
4 ounces no-fat ice cream	¼ honeydew melon	

*100 calories no-fat or low-fat cake, hard candy, cookies, and so forth

*100 calories fruit-based jam, jelly, and so forth

1 ounce raisins or figs

4-ounce can of fruit, unsweetened and in its own juice (no more than one serving per day)

* ½ cup juice

* No more than three or four times a week

Note: The ice cream can also be used in the dairy category.

Limited Complex Carbohydrates: You should have five to seven servings a day.

One serving consists of the following:

BREADS, CEREALS, GRAINS

½ bagel

2 slices low-fat whole wheat bread

1 English muffin

8 low-fat or no-fat crackers

4 rice cakes

1 pita bread

1 ounce cold cereal

1 ounce hot cereal (before cooking)

VEGETABLES

1 large baked potato

¾ cup jerusalem artichoke

1 medium sweet potato or yam

1 cup corn kernels

1 large corn on the cob

½ cup beans or lentils of any kind (used also as a protein)

1 cup peas of any kind

⅔ cup pasta, cooked	1 cup beets
⅔ cup rice, cooked	1 large acorn (winter) squash
½ cup barley, cooked	3 cups popcorn made with no oil
1 ounce pretzels	

Note: If you cook your pasta *al dente*, it behaves as a complex carbohydrate, so don't worry that it will behave as a sugar and retard your ability to burn fat.

Unlimited Complex Carbohydrates: Minimum of six servings a day. One serving consists of ½ cup cooked or 1 cup raw, unless otherwise specified, of the following:

Asparagus	Lettuce
Beans, green or yellow	Mushrooms
Broccoli	Okra
Cabbage, Chinese cabbage	Onions
Carrots	Parsnips
Cauliflower	Peppers, green or red
Celery	Radishes
Chicory	Rutabagas
Collard greens	Shallots
Cucumber	Spinach
Eggplant	Sprouts
Endive	Squash (summer or zucchini)
Escarole	Tomatoes
Frozen mixed vegetables	Turnips
Kale	Vegetable juice (6 ounces)*
Leeks	

* No more than two servings a day. (You need the fiber from the actual vegetables.)

Fiber: Why It's Important and Where You Will Get It

Fiber helps prevent colon cancer and a host of other diseases, but in addition it aids in the removal of fat from your digestive system. Here's how it works: When fiber leaves your body through elimination, some of the fat in your digestive system clings to the rough surface of the fiber and is pulled along with it. In this sense, fiber behaves as a "fat vacuum."

Fiber falls into two categories: soluble and insoluble. Soluble fiber is found in oat bran, psyllium, fresh fruits and vegetables, and legumes. This type of fiber can be digested by the body when consumed. It helps lower blood sugar and cholesterol levels. Insoluble fiber is found in whole wheat, whole grains, celery, corn, bran, green beans, green leafy vegetables, potato skins, and brown rice. This type of fiber cannot be digested by the body. About 15 percent of a food with this type of fiber is automatically eliminated, and in that sense the calorie count of these foods is really 15 percent less than you think. Insoluble fiber provides the stool with needed volume and helps prevent constipation and colon and rectal cancer.

You need about 30 grams of fiber a day, but, fortunately, you will automatically get that if you are eating unlimited amounts of complex carbohydrates and some breads and cereals. (There are 8 grams of fiber in one cup of broccoli, for example.)

Dairy: You should have two to three servings a day. One serving consists of the following:

1 glass of skim or 1% fat milk

8 ounces no-fat or 1% yogurt

4 ounces no-fat or 1% cottage cheese

2 tablespoons no-fat or 1% cream cheese

1½ ounces low-fat or no-fat cheese

½ cup low-fat or no-fat ice cream (no more than two or three times a week)

Water and Sodium: Let's Clear It Up Once and for All!

Drinking water does not cause you to retain water; in fact, it helps flush the water from your system. In addition, water cleanses the internal organs and helps the skin look young. More than half of our body weight is water. We could live for a month without eating, but we could survive only a few days without water because we lose three quarts of water a day through perspiration and excretion. In addition, water is the basis of all body fluids, including digestive juices, blood, urine, lymph, and perspiration, and is the main carrier of nutrients throughout the body.

Water is so important to your body that your body will get it one way or another. If you don't drink it, and your body needs water, your body will drive you to eat since most foods contain about 70 percent water.

How much water should you drink? Six to eight eight-ounce glasses a day are recommended. One way is to have a glass in the morning and before each meal and snack, and one before bed. Extra water can be drunk before and after exercising—even during exercising. I have recently changed my water drinking habits. (I drink about ten glasses of water a day!) I am amazed at what it has done for my skin. I also have fewer problems with bloating and water retention. I'm absolutely amazed.

Now what about salt or sodium? Sodium is a much needed mineral. If your body is deprived of sodium, the acid-alkali balance is disturbed and your muscles begin to cramp. Why then do we fear salt? It holds fifty times its own weight in water, so when we consume too much of it, we retain water. How much is too much? Although the USDA says 2,400 milligrams is just fine, it's better to keep it a little lower—about 1,500 to 2,000 milligrams, if possible.

What should you do if you retain water and want to get rid of it? Simple. Drink lots of water and also cut down your sodium to 1,500 milligrams a day. In five days you will have flushed out any excess water. The scale could go down five or more pounds, but you should realize that you lost excess water weight, not fat. On the other hand, if you should gain three or more pounds in a day, realize that it's water retention and not fat. Actually, it's physically impossible to gain that much fat weight in one day.

Where will you get your salt? In the foods you eat. Even lettuce has some sodium (4 milligrams a cup). There are 602 milligrams in six ounces of flounder and 48 milligrams in a cantaloupe. A pickle has a whopping 930 milligrams, and most canned soups have 1,000 milligrams a serving. What does all this mean? Avoid pickled and canned items. You'll get your sodium during the day without trying. And throw away that salt shaker (there are 500 milligrams of sodium in a quarter teaspoon of salt—a few good shakes).

Having said this, I must admit that my body craves sodium—perhaps because my blood pressure is very low. Maybe my body is telling me to have more sodium to raise it a little. I do retain water when I indulge in high-sodium foods, but whenever I cut it, I lose the water weight. I have enough trouble worrying about overeating foods—and gaining fat-weight that doesn't go away in a few days. So I'm not going to obsess about retaining a little water that I can get rid of any time I want by simply cutting my sodium and drinking lots of water.

What About the Other "Bad Guys," Caffeine and Alcohol?

For many, a cup of coffee in the morning provides a needed energy boost to start the day. But is it harmful? The reputation of caffeine changes from day to day. For now, the general consensus in the medical community is to keep your caffeine intake down to a limited amount—no more than three cups of coffee a day, for instance.

There are some potential problems with caffeine. It tends to increase fibro-cystic breast tissue and can aggravate the condition called "cystic breasts." In addition, it can cause rapid heartbeat and, as mentioned above, if consumed in excess, can hinder your body's ability to absorb calcium.

Be aware that caffeine is not found only in coffee (125 milligrams in a brewed cup, 85 milligrams in instant) but in tea and cocoa (35 milligrams a cup) and cola (50 milligrams a glass).

Now let's talk about alcohol. Alcohol functions in the body the same as a simple carbohydrate, so you can substitute it (not more than three times a week) for something in the fruit category. Four ounces of wine or champagne, twelve ounces of beer, or 1½ ounces of hard liquor is equivalent to one serving. Why didn't I include it in the list? I don't want to encourage you to use it because alcohol tends to cause you to let down your guard, and you may decide to "just pick" and break your new eating plan. In addition, alcohol is a relaxant, and slows down your metabolism slightly.

It's a better idea to forgo drinking or at least keep it very limited until you reach your weight goal.

Maintaining Your Weight

Speaking of your weight goal, and before I put the weight loss plan together for you, let me tell you how you will maintain your weight loss forever. You will continue to eat exactly as in this chapter forever! Don't kill me now. There's more to it. You will have two choices: You will be able to either eat anything you want once a week all day long or eat a small something every day. I'll call them plans A and B.

With plan A you get to eat about 20 percent more than you ate when you were dieting—every day. For example, say you ate about 1,500 calories a day to lose the weight. Now you can add 300 calories a day—a total of 1,800 calories—and not gain weight. And those calories can be from any food you choose. For example, now that I found the small boxes of Cheez-It crackers, I eat them. A box is 290 calories, and even though it has 15 grams of fat, I indulge. I do this two or three times a week. Other days I have a juicy cheesy piece of pizza or a heaping amount of full-fat cream cheese on my bagel with lox. Of course, you will have to check with your doctor as to what kinds of fat you can eat.

Plan B is the one I used all the time. You can save extra calories all week and use them in one free eating day. In this case you get to eat about 2,100 extra calories, or a total of 3,600 calories. You can have a juicy steak, chocolate chip cookies, a huge bowl of pasta with lots of sauce—the works. Again, you will have to check with your doctor, but no matter what, you can have the extra calories in this manner in plan A or B and not gain weight once you reach your goal.

But what happens if you find yourself cheating—and eating more than you should on plan A or B, and you start gaining weight? Simple: As soon as you gain more than two or three pounds, don't take advantage of plan A or B until you lose them. I've been doing that, and it is amazing. I've kept my weight "photo-shoot perfect" for over a year now just by doing this. In other words, I no longer gain seven pounds off season and then have to suffer to get them off. I love it. This is a wonderful plan.

Sample Daily Meal Plan

Now for the challenge of putting it all together. Your goal is to consume 15 to 25 grams of fat, two to three portions of protein, two to three portions of dairy, two to four portions of fruit, five to seven portions of limited complex carbohydrates, and at least six servings of unlimited complex carbohydrates. You will keep your sodium under 2,000 milligrams and your calcium intake where it should be, say, 1,500 milligrams. All the while, you will keep your calories around 1,300 to 1,700 (an average of about 1,500 a day) so you can lose weight quickly and safely.

A SAMPLE MEAL PLAN

BREAKFAST

⅔ cup 40% bran flakes cereal	90 calories, 0 fat
1 glass 1% fat milk	100 calories, 2.6 fat grams, 300 milligrams calcium
1½ cups sliced strawberries	69 calories, 0 fat

SNACK

1 cup plain, no-fat yogurt	100 calories, 0 fat, 452 milligrams calcium

LUNCH

1 cup broccoli, cooked from frozen	52 calories, 0 fat, 100 milligrams calcium
2 slices whole wheat bread	80 calories, 1 gram fat
1 ounce mozzarella cheese (part skim)	80 calories, 4.5 grams fat, 207 milligrams calcium
1 medium tomato	26 calories, 0 fat

SNACK

1 medium apple	80 calories, 1 gram fat
1 cup cauliflower	25 calories, 0 fat

DINNER

Chicken breast	180 calories, 4.5 grams fat
1 cup collard greens, cooked from raw	65 calories, 357 milligrams calcium
½ grapefruit	46 calories, 0 fat
1 baked potato	220 calories, 0 fat

SNACK

2 ounces pretzels	200 calories, 2 grams fat

TOTALS:

Calories: 1,413

Fat: 16 grams

Calcium: 1,500 milligrams

Notice that you have followed your required guidelines for protein, dairy, simple and complex carbohydrates—limited and unlimited. You had yogurt, mozzarella cheese, and chicken for your protein. You had yogurt and skim milk for your dairy. You had yogurt, 1 percent milk, mozzarella cheese, and collard greens for your calcium requirement. You had bran flakes, whole wheat bread, a potato, and pretzels for your limited complex carbohydrates. You had broccoli, tomato, cauliflower, and collard greens for your unlimited complex carbohydrates. You had strawberries, an apple, and grapefruit for your fruit.

This is just an example. Make your own meals. This is a review or a guideline. You might also obtain a copy of my book *Eat to Trim*, which includes a whole month's worth of meal plans! (See Bibliography, page 193.)

Note: You can make it easy on yourself by substituting the foods in the above plan with foods in the same categories. Don't think that anything has to be eaten specifically at any meal. You can switch the meals around, too. Lunch could be breakfast, and dinner could be lunch. The snacks can be reversed or added to lunches, and some lunches can be used for snacks. Have fun. But spread your food around. Don't go more than three or four hours without eating, and eat at least five times a day. Otherwise, your metabolism will slow down, and you won't burn as much fat! Happy eating!

If you have any questions or comments, please write to me at my address below, but be sure to include a stamped, self-addressed envelope if you want a reply.

Joyce L. Vedral
P.O. Box 7433
Wantagh, NY 11793-7433

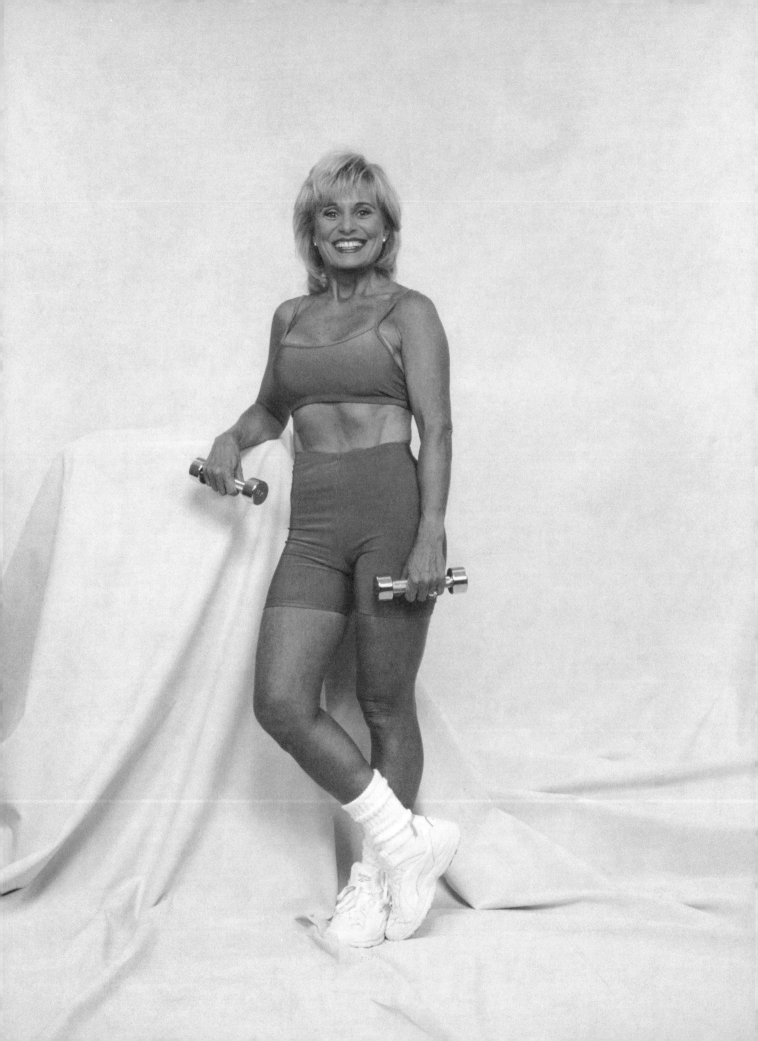

Notes

Chapter 1: Build Bone, Strengthen Muscle, and Create a Beautiful Body in the Bargain

1. Brown, Susan E., Ph.D., *Better Bones, Better Body*. New Canaan, CT: Keats Publishing, 1996, pp. 145–46.

2. Pruitt, L.A., et al., "Weight-Training Effects on Bone Mineral Density in Early Postmenopausal Women." *Journal of Bone and Mineral Research* 7: 2 (February 1992): 179–85.

3. Notelovitz, M., et al., "Estrogen Therapy and Variable-Resistance Weight Training Increase Bone Mineral in Surgically Menopausal Women." *Journal of Bone and Mineral Research* 6: 6 (June 1991): 583–90. Two groups of menopausal women were given estrogen, but only one group was allowed to work out with weights. At the end of one year, the women taking estrogen alone maintained but did not increase bone density. The women doing the weight training significantly increased the bone density of not only the spine but also the forearm. "The results of this study show that variable-resistance training in estrogen-replete women adds bone to both the axial and appendicular skeleton."

4. Brown, Susan E., Ph.D., *Better Bones, Better Body*, pp. 227–28. Brown lists various studies which prove that weight training not only halted but reversed osteoporosis of women ranging in age from their forties through their seventies.

5. Ruth S. Jacobowitz, *150 Most-Asked Questions About Osteoporosis*. New York: Hearst Books, 1993, p. 115.

6. Miriam E. Nelson, Ph.D., *Strong Women Stay Young*. New York: Bantam Books, 1997, p. 5.

7. Ruth S. Jacobowitz, *150 Most-Asked Questions*, p. 117.

8. Wayne L. Prescott, Ph.D., "Strength Training Update." *Idea Today* (June 1995), p. 1.

9. Miriam E. Nelson, Ph.D., *Strong Women Stay Young*, pp. 63, 66. Nelson is talking about her own mother-in-law! She points out that this is definitely not an activity she would recommend for a woman in her late seventies who has had a hip fracture.

Chapter 2: Bone in the Bank

1. Heinonen, A., et al., "Bone Mineral Density of Female Athletes in Different Sports." *Bone Miner* 23: 1 (October 1993): 1–14. Groups of women in various endurance sports, including a group of weight-training women, were measured for bone density and then remeasured after six months. Only the weight trainers had a significant increase in bone density at the lumbar spine, distal femur, patella, proximal tibia, and distal radius. The conclusion of the study was that weight training provides more effective osteogenic stimulus than endurance training.

2. Susan E. Brown, Ph.D., *Better Bones, Better Body*. New Canaan, CT: Keats Publishing, 1996, p. 320.

3. Ibid., p. 66.

4. Ibid., p. 145.

5. Jane E. Brody, "Can Exercise Prevent Breast Cancer?" *The New York Times*, May 12, 1997, p. C12.

6. Ibid., p. 144. "Exercise builds bone at all ages. It is absolutely essential for optimum bone development in the young, and without it aging bone regeneration is limited. Nutrition alone cannot bring about maximum peak bone mass or maintain optimum bone mass as we age. Exercise is not optional."

7. Miriam E. Nelson, Ph.D., *Strong Women Stay Young*. New York: Bantam Books, 1997, pp. 37–38.

8. Ibid., p. 73.

Bibliography

Joyce Vedral Books

Weight Training Made Easy: From Beginner to Expert in Four Simple Steps. New York: Warner Books, 1997.

Eat to Trim. Warner Books, 1997.

Definition: Shape Without Bulk in Fifteen Minutes a Day. New York: Warner Books, 1995.

Top Shape. New York: Warner Books, 1995.

The College Dorm Workout. With Marthe S. Vedral. New York: Warner Books, 1994.

Bottoms Up! New York: Warner Books, 1993.

Gut Busters. New York: Warner Books, 1992.

The Fat-Burning Workout. New York: Warner Books, 1991.

The 12-Minute Total-Body Workout. New York: Warner Books, 1989.

Now or Never. New York: Warner Books, 1986.

Joyce Vedral Self-Help Books

Look In, Look Up—Look Out!! Be the Person You Were Meant to Be. New York: Warner Books, 1996.

Get Rid of Him. New York: Warner Books, 1993.

Joyce Vedral Videos

The Bottoms Up Workout: Upper Body. New York: Good Times Video, 1995.

The Bottoms Up Workout: Middle Body. New York: Good Times Video, 1995.

The Bottoms Up Workout: Lower Body. New York: Good Times Video, 1995.

The Fat-Burning Workout, Volume 1 (The Regular Workout), 1993. A-Vision videos.

The Fat-Burning Workout, Volume 2 (The Intensity and Insanity Workout), 1993. A-Vision videos.

Please write to me (see page 189) if you can't find any of my books or videos, or if you have any questions or comments. Enclose a stamped, self-addressed envelope, and I'll personally answer your letter. Remember, we are in this together.

INDEX

Appendix

Tear-Out Chart

Here is an Exercise-at-a-Glance easy reference chart to hang on your wall and make your workout even easier. Just cut along the dotted lines, tape to a wall in your exercise area, and get going!

Back and Abdominal Workout: Warm-Ups

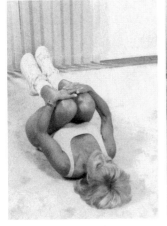

BACK PRESS KNEE RAISE: START

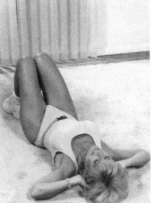

BACK PRESS KNEE RAISE: FINISH

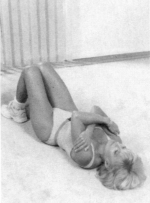

DINOSAUR CURL: START

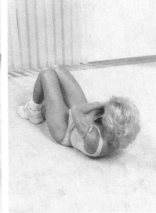

DINOSAUR CURL: FINISH

Back Exercises

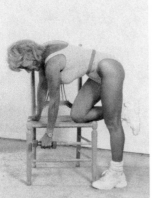

LEANING ONE-ARM DUMBBELL ROW: START

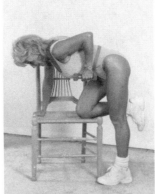

LEANING ONE-ARM DUMBBELL ROW: FINISH

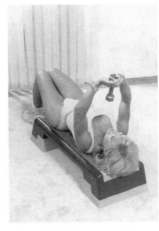

BACK OVERHEAD PULLOVER: START

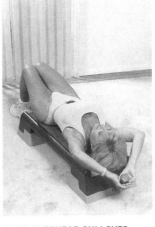

BACK OVERHEAD PULLOVER: FINISH

Abdominal Exercises

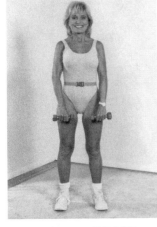

DOUBLE-ARM UPRIGHT ROW: START

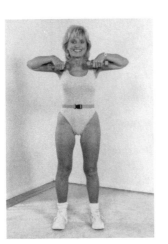

DOUBLE-ARM UPRIGHT ROW: FINISH

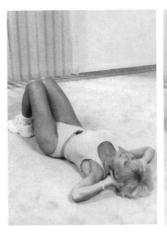

CRUNCH: START

CRUNCH: FINISH

Abdominal Exercises (cont'd)

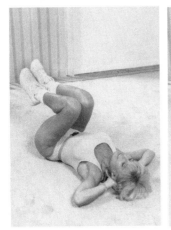

BENT-KNEE SEWN LIFT: START

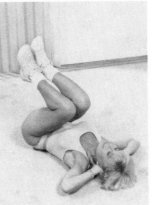

BENT-KNEE SEWN LIFT: FINISH

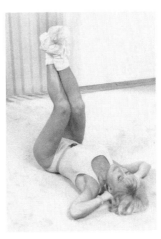

CEILING LIFT: START

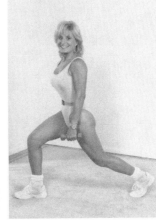

CEILING LIFT: FINISH

Leg and Hip/Buttocks Workout: Warm-Ups

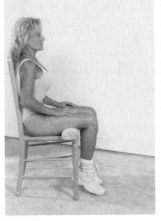

SINGLE LEG EXTENSION: START

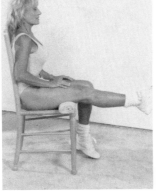

SINGLE LEG EXTENSION: FINISH

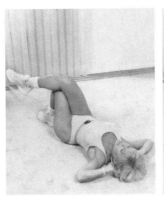

LYING CROSSOVER: START

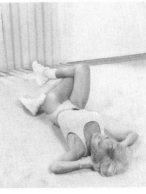

LYING CROSSOVER: FINISH

Leg Exercises

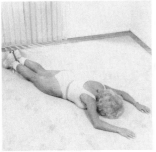

LEG CURL: START

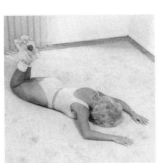

LEG CURL: FINISH

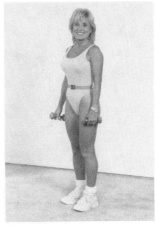

LUNGE: START

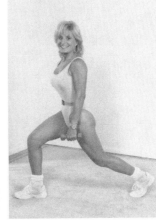

LUNGE: FINISH

Leg Exercises (cont'd)

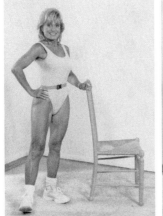

INNER THIGH SWEEP: START

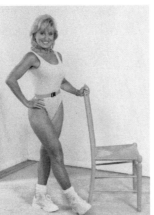

INNER THIGH SWEEP: FINISH

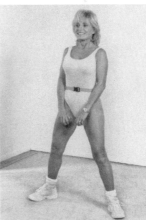

ALT: WIDE LEG SEMI-SQUAT: START

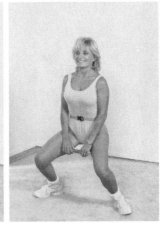

WIDE LEG SEMI-SQUAT: FINISH

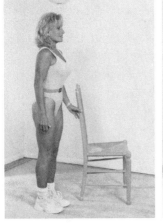

STANDING CALF RAISE: START

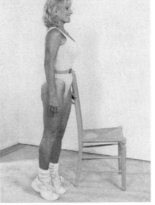

STANDING CALF RAISE: FINISH

Hip/Buttocks Exercises

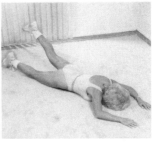

ALTERNATE PRONE BUTT LIFT: START

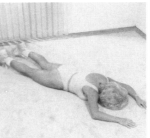

ALTERNATE PRONE BUTT LIFT: FINISH

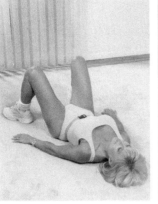

LYING BUTT LIFT: START

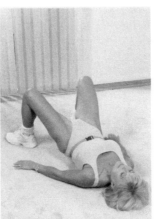

LYING BUTT LIFT: FINISH

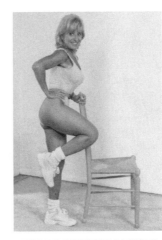

STANDING BENT-KNEE BACK LEG EXTENSION: START

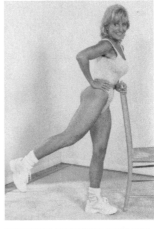

STANDING BENT-KNEE BACK LEG EXTENSION: FINISH

Arms: Wrist, Biceps, Triceps Workout: Warm-Ups

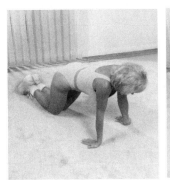

DOGGIE PAW WRIST-FOREARM STRETCH: START

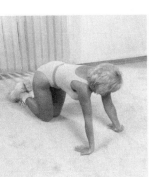

DOGGIE PAW WRIST-FOREARM STRETCH: FINISH

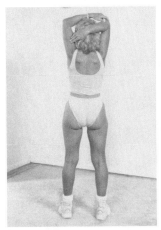

SCRATCH-YOUR-BACK BICEPS-TRICEPS PULL: START

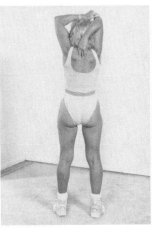

SCRATCH-YOUR-BACK BICEPS-TRICEPS PULL: FINISH

Wrist Exercises

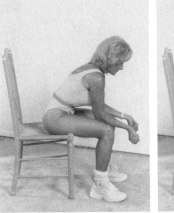

PALMS-UP WRIST CURL: START

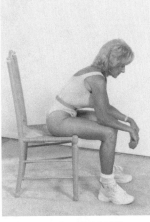

PALMS-UP WRIST CURL: FINISH

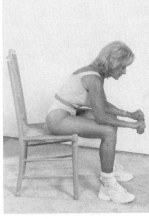

PALMS-DOWN WRIST RAISE: START

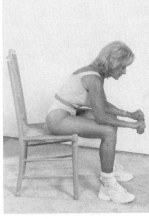

PALMS-DOWN WRIST RAISE: FINISH

Biceps Exercises

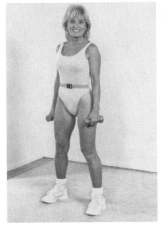

STANDING SIMULTANEOUS CURL: START

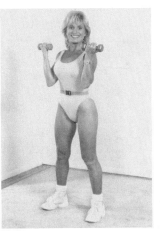

STANDING SIMULTANEOUS CURL: FINISH

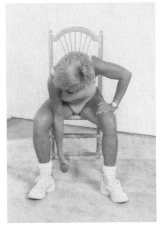

CONCENTRATION CURL: START

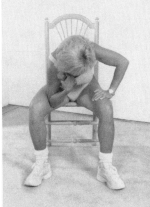

CONCENTRATION CURL: FINISH

Triceps Exercises

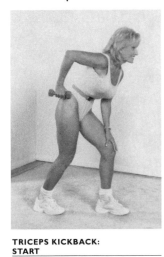

TRICEPS KICKBACK: START

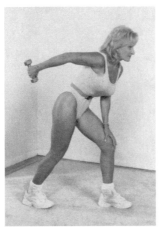

TRICEPS KICKBACK: FINISH

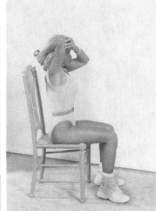

SEATED ONE-ARM OVERHEAD EXTENSION: START

SEATED ONE-ARM OVERHEAD EXTENSION: FINISH

Shoulder and Chest Workout: Warm-Ups

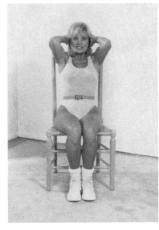

HUG-YOUR-HEAD SHOULDER-BACK STRETCH: START

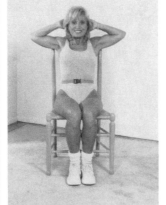

HUG-YOUR-HEAD SHOULDER-BACK STRETCH: FINISH

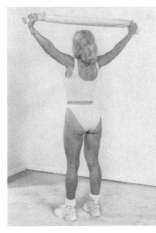

OVERHEAD TOWEL CHEST STRETCH: START

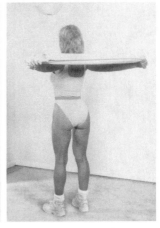

OVERHEAD TOWEL CHEST STRETCH: FINISH

Shoulder Exercises

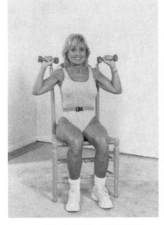

SEATED SIMULTANEOUS DUMB-BELL PRESS: START

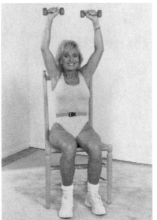

SEATED SIMULTANEOUS DUMB-BELL PRESS: FINISH

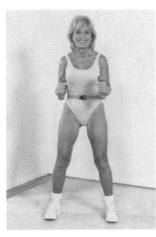

EASY-DOES-IT SIDE LATERAL: START

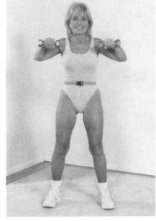

EASY-DOES-IT SIDE LATERAL: FINISH

Shoulder Exercises (cont'd)

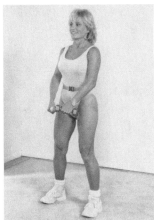

ALT: REGULAR SIDE LATERAL: START

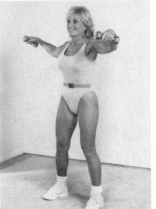

REGULAR SIDE LATERAL: FINISH

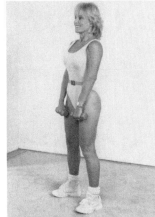

ALTERNATE FRONT RAISE: START

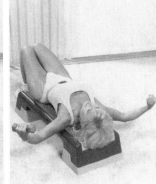

ALTERNATE FRONT RAISE: FINISH

Chest Exercises

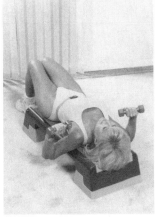

DUMBBELL BENCH PRESS: START

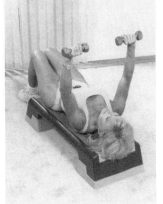

DUMBBELL BENCH PRESS: FINISH

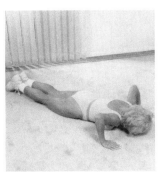

EASY-DOES-IT PUSH-UP: START

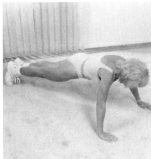

EASY-DOES-IT PUSH-UP: FINISH

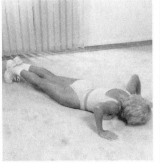

ALT: REGULAR PUSH-UP: START

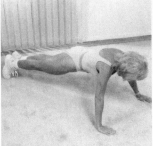

REGULAR PUSH-UP: FINISH

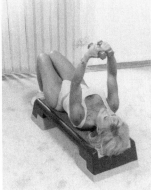

DUMBBELL FLY: START

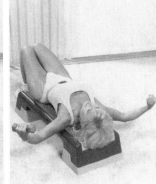

DUMBBELL FLY: FINISH